Full Heart
Satisfied Belly

Full Heart
Satisfied Belly

by
Kathleen S. Hosner, Ph.D.
and
Linda Frazee

iUniverse, Inc.
New York Lincoln Shanghai

Full Heart Satisfied Belly

iUniverse, Inc.

For information address:
iUniverse, Inc.
2021 Pine Lake Road, Suite 100
Lincoln, NE 68512
www.iuniverse.com

Throughout this book, the authors have used real-life case examples from their respective practices. The names cited and quoted have been changed throughout in order to ensure their clients' anonymity.
The theories and formulae presented in this book are expressed as the authors' opinions and are not intended in any manner whatsoever to diagnose, prescribe, or administer to any physical or mental ailments. In all matters regarding health, readers are directed to contact a qualified, licensed health practitioner.

ISBN: 0-595-31757-X

Printed in the United States of America

We dedicate this to the child in all of us that desires the freedom to feel fully satiated with life, and especially to our children and grandchildren: Leigha, Elizabeth, Brennan, Raymond, Michael Byran, Michelle, Brad, Jesse, Noel, Jaden, Christian, Antonette, Danyelle, and Michael Steven.

Contents

Part II

Part III

Acknowledgments

To our husbands, Frank and Richard, for their patience, support and computer skills during this growing experience

and

to Hilda Villaverde for introducing us and igniting the spark of this book as a possibility.

and

for professional and technical support and the encouraging words that kept the project moving, we would like to acknowledge:

Diane Cummings
Sherry Folb
Paul M. Howey
Kathy Evans Peters
Robert and Jeanne Petrick
Karen Sheehan
Jayn Stewart

From Kathleen, in gratitude to Virginia Jenkins who taught me to trust my inner wisdom and helped me touch into my body's innate wisdom to heal.

From Linda, with gratitude to my friend Jo Sherrill who was my first co-facilitator and teacher of this material.

And we thank our clients, for they have all inspired us and been our teachers.

Preface

Kathleen Hosner, Ph.D., has been in the health care industry for 30 years. Her years of experience led her from one facet of medicine to the next. Starting as a nurse then a Physician Assistant she enjoyed the interaction of patients and loved the study of the body and the wondrous way it works that went along with it. After having two daughters she found she needed regular business hours to be an involved parent. This led her to going back to school and getting her M.S. in Health Administration. She then spent ten years in an administrative position with a busy physician practice and large medical center.

It took a life threatening bout with hepatitis that introduced her to alternative and ancient ways of practicing medicine. Her curiosity got the best of her and she was eager to learn why these ways worked. She returned to school and received her Ph.D. in Nutrition. She started her own private practice in Scottsdale, Arizona to help others as she had been helped. She started teaching people how to listen to their inner guidance and body for the wisdom to heal and feel good, which was well received. People always wanted more and kept asking her to write a book. So in response, *Full Heart/Satisfied Belly* was written. It is with passion, spirit, and heart that she has poured *her all* into this book to give back what she has received—the goal, so that others may live abundantly.

Linda Frazee was born in the 1940's, and both her parents were deeply affected by the depression and deprivation due to poverty. Throughout her childhood there was an undertone of there not being enough of everything, especially food. In addition, her father disapproved of how much her mother weighed. Her mother was a brilliant and beautiful woman but seldom ever felt that truth. Instead her life satisfaction was diminished by the fifteen pounds she lost and gained over and over again.

Linda inherited her mother's body style and many of the feelings she had about herself. Her struggles with food and weight began when she was a teenager. She unconsciously tied her self-image to the 10 or 15 pounds she lost repeatedly to be good enough. Even after discovering high-quality food, she continued to eat emotionally. Instead of facing some of her tough life issues, she was out of touch with the still, small voice inside that knew why she was eating. In her case it took a divorce, facing her workaholic behavior, and learning to go within to listen for guidance before she began to have peace with her body.

As a transpersonal therapist she has worked with thousands of individuals about the drain of life energy that occurs when we don't love our bodies. She has a thriving private practice in Scottsdale, Arizona, helping people accept their bodies as a gift.

Linda wrote this book for her mother and her generation, the women of her own generation, her daughters, granddaughter and every woman who has ever felt less than because of the way her body looks.

I

Introduction

A small child sits paralyzed at the dinner table while his parents scream and shout at each other. A beautiful teenager rushes to the bathroom to vomit the lunch she just ate with her friends at school. A hardworking husband and father, who had coffee and donuts for breakfast on his way to the office, a take-out burger for lunch, and a diet cola on his way to the gym after work. Examples such as these are being played out every day by millions of people across America. It's people such as these that the authors see in their private practices.

With little or no success, the authors' clients have tried countless ways to improve their nutrition, to stop their various addictions, and to resolve their childhood traumas. What these people all have in common is a deep hunger that never seems to be filled. This craving, which is often misinterpreted as a hunger for food, is instead a craving to be connected to one's own body and emotions, to other human beings, to the earth, and most of all to one's spirit.

In the space of just one or two generations, our society has moved from one of "connectedness" to one of isolation and separateness. We no longer have the comfort and reassurance of an extended family to teach us about growing and preparing our food and about celebrating our interconnectedness as a family each evening at dinner. We have lost our connection to the earth and the food it so lovingly yields to nourish us. The connectivity of our extended families has been replaced by long work hours, television shows, and busy schedules. Children today see their parents take their dinners out of the freezer and pop them into the microwave. Often the whole family stares at the television set as they eat, more connected to some TV drama than to one another.

Our children have come to believe our food comes from the grocery store instead of the nurturing earth. Today, families are more focused on technology than on each other. With all this has come an enormous and not-so-subtle cost to our emotional, spiritual, and physical health—a cost that no one ever anticipated.

Long ago, there was a time when your grandmother used to know what backyard herb would heal your tummy ache. It was a time when the family doctor who delivered you, came to know your whole physical and emotional history, and would visit you in your home to administer whatever healing in whatever form was needed. Granted, he may have been limited by a lack of technology and diagnostic tools, but his loving touch and the knowledge that your body possesses the innate wisdom to heal was often all that was needed. His greatest gifts were those of intuitive knowledge and an understanding of the natural processes of disease and healing.

Contrast that with today's world. Mary has had a recurring headache for the past several weeks which has proved to be more than just a nuisance to learning her new high-stress job and adjusting to her transfer to Chicago. It was only after she grabbed an empty bottle of extra-strength aspirin that she realized how many pills she had taken in a relatively short period of time without the benefit of any relief. She didn't even attempt to discover whatever factors may have been causing her headaches. As a last resort, she looked in her new HMO benefits book to find a physician with hours and a location that were convenient to her hectic schedule. The doctor she chose took a history, gave her a preliminary physical, and prescribed a headache medication. It never occurred to either one of them to consider whether Mary's anxiety about her new job, the loneliness of her new life in a new city, or her predominantly fast-food diet could be contributing to her frequent headaches.

It is time to become connected to our birthright: the power to have healthy bodies that we honor and respect for the miraculous abilities they afford us. So how do we become connected? The first step is to identify the ways we disconnect in our present lives. For example, have you ever sat in front of your computer so long that your legs went to sleep because you failed to recognize your body's need for movement? Have you ever gone from sunup to bedtime and had little or no recollection of what you'd eaten all day? Do you tend to ignore a sore throat until it turns into a full-blown cold? Do you find yourself saying you're fine when, in all honesty, you are really furious inside? Do you prefer to distract yourself by keeping busy rather than truly feeling some particular emotional pain or loss? When you are afraid, do you clam up? Or do you find yourself lashing out at others?

It's possible that you might not recognize any of the above as symptoms of disconnection because in our society, they are commonly accepted as normal. Keep in mind, however, that "normal" is neither necessarily healthy nor satisfying. To question our society's norm of "disconnectedness," you have to be willing to challenge old patterns and long-held beliefs. Also, you'll have to stop blaming others for your circumstances, your shortcomings, and your aches, pains, and stress.

Amazing things happen when you leave behind your feelings of victimization and choose to be responsible for your life. Learning to tap into your inner wisdom, instead of always relying on outside authority, opens up a whole world of unlimited possibilities. You will experience new feelings that ultimately will translate into new life behaviors.

Did you know that your thoughts, emotions, and beliefs have energy that are responsible for creating your reality? Since energy and matter are one and the same thing, and energy vibrates at different frequencies—the lower the vibrations or frequencies, the more dense the energy becomes. It is the density of energy that determines whether we can see something with our human eye or hear it with our ear. Just because we can't see or hear something is not proof that it doesn't exist. It just means that it is vibrating at a frequency beyond our ability to physically perceive it. Therefore, because we are all energy, we are each connected to all other living things.

In truth, it is impossible to be disconnected from any part of yourself (even though that is a common illusion). Thoughts, emotions, and words are also all energy, oscillating through our world at whatever vibration with which we send them out. It is also commonly accepted that like attracts like. For example, when we send forth low vibrations of fear in the form of guilt, loneliness, anger, resentment, worry, doubt, frustration, stress, and confusion, then we have invited those same emotions/vibrations to return to us. By this process, we keep perpetuating the same things that made us feel bad in the first place. If others around us are also creating fear-based thoughts and emotions, the resulting synergy forms a collective belief that we are separate and disconnected.

The good news is that you can change all this. You can learn to create happiness and health in your own life by defining what you want and by using your thoughts and emotions to create it. You will be generating thought patterns that vibrate at higher levels. These higher energy levels will resonate more closely with who you really are—the life essence connected to the very source of life. As a result, you will be vibrating at a frequency that creates ever greater and greater possibilities. It is in this space that you will no longer be hungry, for you will have become very connected and very full.

Our thoughts are patterned after beliefs we've established in the past either consciously or unconsciously. Part I of this book will help you identify the myths around the beliefs (and, therefore, the thoughts) about food that we have as individuals and as a society. Food is something to which we all relate several times a day, every day. By connecting to our inner wisdom and our ability to create health in the area of food, we will learn how to create improved health in all other areas of our lives.

Our spirit, our mind, and our body are one. They are not disjointed parts, as the separateness way of thinking has led us to believe. They can either vibrate in harmony as a finely tuned instrument making beautiful music or they can vibrate discordantly and create offensive sounds that manifest themselves as dissatisfaction, disease, and dysfunctional relationships. The choice is ours.

In Part I, we provide you with the tools to make peace with your body and through that peace to find deep satisfaction in eating. Our goal is not to give you another diet book, but to teach you how to trust your inner wisdom and become your own authority concerning what you eat, how much, and why. In other words, we will present you with a holistic approach to your relationship with food. We will help you to *think for one minute* before you decide to eat something, putting yourself on a behavioral path toward *feeling good for a lifetime.* We want you *to make peace with your body,* to be satiated with life—in other words, to have a *Full Heart/Satisfied Belly.*

1

The Tangled Web of Food and Love

Somewhere at this exact moment a baby is being born. Once safely out of the womb, its primary objective will be to suckle at its mother's breast. Without that strong drive, the human race would perish. Eating and suckling are vital ways a newborn feels comfort, safety, and hopefully love. From the moment of birth, the emotional connection between love and food is so intertwined that separating them is almost impossible.

That simple bond is so basic and so natural that ideally we would respond to our adult selves as easily as a loving mother to her new child. Our bodies are designed to communicate to our minds when we are ready to eat and to know exactly what kind of food we need. This exchange of vital information between body and mind is present in every human being. This connection is our birthright.

So what happens to make us feel disconnected from that natural state of being? The answer is complicated and varies from individual to individual. We will begin to trace through life stages some of the key components of experiences that influence us and eventually make us feel disconnected from our body's clear messages about food and eating. As we do so, we ask that you remember this important truth:

Underneath any discontent you may feel with your body are messages of guidance designed to keep you at your highest experience of health. *These messages are always being communicated.* Perhaps you have just forgotten how to listen.

That forgetting to listen may have started soon after you were born. As a baby you were dependent upon your caretakers to know your needs and to meet them. The only way you could communicate at that age was by crying, and crying is easily misinterpreted. Seeds of difficulty can be planted in the child if problems arise with nursing and feeding. Persistent difficulties with nursing, allergies to milk, parent's tension during feeding, and medical problems can all fill the feeding time with stress.

Newborns are highly attuned to the feelings of their parents and caretakers, and they respond to stress in their own ways. When parents or caregivers worry about an infant who is not eating properly or not gaining weight rapidly, the baby internalizes that emotion just as readily and as completely as a sponge absorbs water. A message that something is wrong is sent throughout the child's nervous system. When infants feel uncomfortable for any reason, some may refuse to eat, whereas others may overeat.

In an effort to meet their infant's need, parents turn to the current books, myths, and professional theories of that particular time for guidance. If your baby is having difficulty with feeding and you are worried about it, the most important thing to do is to quiet your own fears. If that's hard to do on your own, get help from a family member, friend, doctor, or another professional who works with children and eating-related problems. It's important to get the support you need in calming any apprehensions you may have regarding your baby's health and well-being.

Infant Eating Patterns Carry Over Into Adulthood

In the past, a prevalent theory asserted that newborns and infants can control and manipulate their parents. Therefore, the theory concludes, their cries of hunger should simply be ignored. Mothers and fathers were told to put their babies on strict feeding schedules that fit the parents' lifestyle. (Some theories still promote this philosophy!) The truth is that since babies are all different from one another, no one system could possibly be appropriate for every child. In Linda's therapy practice, she has worked with many people whose parents followed this practice of strict feeding schedules. As a result, some of these people exhibited exaggerated fears about being hungry and developed eating disorders as adults. Emma, one of Linda's clients, illustrates the connection between infant eating patterns and an adult eating disorder.

As a baby, Emma cried lustily when she was hungry. She needed, indeed she demanded, to be fed. Emma's mother had read the latest book on "training your baby" and therefore believed in strict schedules. Whenever Emma cried, the first thing her mother did was look at her watch and say, "Sorry baby, it's not time for lunch yet." Emma would just continue to cry, becoming more frantic as each minute passed. Her basic survival instinct was screaming to be met. When the "appropriate feeding time" finally arrived, Emma was physically and emotionally starving. She would gulp down her food and eat far more than she needed. Although she wasn't consciously aware of it, Emma had begun to fear that her needs for food and love would never be met. Throughout her infancy, this stressful feeding pattern was repeated over and over. The belief that there was not enough food became locked inside Emma's mind and programmed into the cells of her body.

Forty years later, Emma was still overeating at every meal, unconsciously attempting to feed that crying infant inside her at the expense of her adult body. (She was thirty pounds overweight.) Her fear of being hungry was so prevalent that she was completely out of touch with what true hunger felt like.

How Family Eating Patterns Develop

Behaviors that are passed from one generation to another are called "family patterns." In other words, mom and dad treat their children the same way their own parents treated them, and in the same way their grandparents were treated by their parents before them, all throughout their families of origin.

When parents have their own issues about eating, they unconsciously bring them to their child's feeding time. As in Emma's case, they may have felt deprived of adequate love and food in their own childhood. Without realizing they are overcompensating for this feeling of deprivation, they eat too much at every meal and also overfeed their children. On the other side of the coin, some people grow up in families that do not value or focus much on food, so as adults they are not interested in food either. They eat only to stay alive; meals are just part of the mechanics of living. If these parents have a child who is constantly hungry or interested in food, they may shame the child for this behavior.

Families usually have unspoken rules about how to deal with feelings, and those rules frequently crop up at mealtimes. The most common and unspoken dysfunctional rules are: *don't tell, don't trust*, and *don't feel*. The family meals might be punctuated with tirades where adults display emotional outbursts, shame the children, criticize each other, or create other types of fearful atmosphere. In these situations, strong feelings bubble up within the child, but he knows he'd better not say anything. It takes a lot of energy not to express feelings, and one way to suppress them is to overeat or under eat, or just make comfort food the food of choice.

Another family's meals may be uncomfortable because of silence. Although the parents are obviously angry or sad, they don't talk about what is bothering them. If the children ask what is wrong, the parents deny there is a problem. The children don't know what to do with the apparent conflict between the behaviors they observe and their parents' words. The air is thick with tension. Everyone at the table silently eats more and more, or not at all.

Even the best-intentioned parents can accidentally teach their children to suppress their feelings through overeating or under eating. For example, when mom and dad are having an argument, their toddler Amanda becomes frightened and starts to cry. Unconsciously, mom hands Amanda a bottle of milk even though there is no reason to believe she is hungry. With the nipple in her mouth, the child calms down. Meanwhile, the argument continues. If this behavior occurs regularly, Amanda may develop the habit of comforting herself with food. This behavior frequently shows up in adults as the craving for a specific food (often ice cream) whenever they are in the presence of conflict.

Sometimes food is used to ease a child's pain. Tanner falls down, cuts his knee, and bursts into tears. Hoping to make him feel better, his concerned mother offers him cookies. In other instances, food may be used to occupy a bored child. For instance, little Mollie is tired of playing with her stuffed toys and tries to get her mother's attention. Mom is in the middle of balancing her checkbook and doesn't want to be disturbed, so she gives her daughter a handful of animal crackers to keep her quiet. In and of themselves, these are not destructive behaviors, so long as they happen infrequently. If they become habitual, however, food ends up becoming a substitute for comfort, attention, and love.

Bill and Eileen represent another example of how food can become associated with comfort. Although they often argue with each other at mealtimes, they are on their best behavior on Sundays when the whole family eats at Bill's mother's house. On Sundays then, their children can relax and feel comfortable at their grandmother's. They love the meal she always serves: roast beef, mashed potatoes with gravy, biscuits and butter, applesauce, and creamed peas. Then grandma tops the whole thing off with hot apple pie and vanilla ice cream. Wow, dessert! Warm feelings *and* sweet goodies given to you by someone you love. What could be better? Bob and Eileen's children grow up contrasting the tension-filled moments of their meals at home where they don't like to eat with the cherished memories of those Sunday dinners. Food once again forms the centerpiece of a powerful image of comfort, connection, and safety.

As these examples show, early childhood experiences at mealtimes create strong memories that can interfere with healthy eating habits all the way into adulthood. If family meals are fraught with discomfort, chilly silence, arguments, criticism, or violence, the dinner table is a scary place for the child. Children exposed to traumatic family meals often feel an ache in the pit in their stomach whenever they have to sit with others and eat. By contrast, they feel most comfortable when eating by themselves.

When we are under stress, many of us find ourselves eating foods that remind us of our childhood years. Occasionally reverting to "comfort" foods is a natural thing. But eating a steady diet of these can be a sign that we are not adequately feeling and expressing our emotions. And they can add extra pounds to our bodies.

"A few months ago, I had a car accident," explains Linda, "and, although I was not seriously injured, I was shaken up for a few weeks. During my recovery, I was overwhelmingly attracted to a particular type of crunchy cookies. I ate one of these cookies after lunch for several days in a row. I seldom eat sugar, so that was unusual for me. When I thought about it, I realized I was comforting myself with one of my favorite childhood treats. Even though my behavior surprised me, I allowed myself that 'comfort' food without feeling guilty. As time went by and I became more relaxed about the accident, I no longer wanted this lunchtime treat. If I had still been eating sugar months later, however, I would have needed to address my underlying feelings about wanting sugar before I could successfully let go of my emotional demand for it. If you have a history of craving sugar, just realize that it's difficult to stop eating it." (See "Addictions to Food" later in this chapter.)

Adolescence and Eating Disorders

Although the seeds for unhealthy eating habits are often planted in infancy or childhood, actual eating disorders usually don't appear until adolescence. Two types of common adolescent eating disorders are bulimia and anorexia. The natural insecurities that go with being a teenager—combined with easy access to fast food (with its inherent low nutritional value) and the penchant for substituting food for emotional expression—can create a host of problems for teens.

If you are the parent of a teenager who is seriously overweight or underweight, you need to know that the situation is not actually about food. Overeating and under eating are generally symptoms of a deeper problem, usually the feeling that your adolescent feels that his or her life is somehow out of control. The unsure teenager needs to feel in charge of *something*, and eating seems to be the easiest thing to control. Adolescence is often when young people begin to feel disconnected from their developing body. For some, anorexia or bulimia unfortunately fills that void. So you see, simply trying to put a teenager on a diet or trying to force-feed him/her won't produce lasting results.

How do you handle the situation? First, deal with your own fears. What are *you* most afraid of? In attempting to help your children, you could create more problems by projecting your own fears onto them. Your challenge will be to learn how to express your feelings, understand your own relationship with food, set clear emotional and psychological boundaries for yourself, clarify important relationships, and address other important issues in your life. (If you feel you are unable to do this on your own, you may wish to seek out a support group to help you on your path.)

How able are you to comfort and support your teenager at this time? Your child may need a therapist and a supportive group setting, especially if anorexic or bulimic, where he or she can talk with other adolescents who are dealing with similar issues. Now here's the hard part: don't overreact, but don't put your head in the sand, either. That's why as a parent you may need outside assistance to understand the situation and keep your emotional balance.

Addictions to Food

While we understand how eating patterns develop, it's not difficult to see why food is the number one addiction in America. It's legal, it's easily accessible, and it satisfies us deeply (particularly on emotional levels). Most of us have no idea how emotionally heavy-laden the simple act of eating is. Rather than feel, we eat. When we are faced with a difficult decision, we eat. Food is a trusted friend that never talks back. It's dependable and it's always available.

As with all addictions, however, the "substance" doesn't come without the physical, emotional, and spiritual consequences that are commonly associated with all addictions. And, as is the case with other addictions, the amount we ingest has to be increased over time to give us the "high"—or satisfaction—it once did. If eating is our only pleasure, it's no wonder we overdo it!

Janet's situation is a perfect example. Her childhood "comfort" food was glazed donuts. As an adult, she learned that donuts had no nutritional value and that the refined sugar in them in fact harmed her body. So she vowed to give up donuts, and she kept her commitment to herself for ten years. Then her marriage began to crumble. At first, Janet allowed herself a treat of one donut with her coffee before work on Fridays, rationalizing that she had been altogether too strict with herself regarding her "no donuts" pledge. As tension in her marriage escalated, she began eating a donut every day. She told herself that these were hard times and one donut a day wasn't going to kill anybody.

On the day she discovered her husband was having an affair, she bought twelve donuts and ate them all in one sitting. It didn't help. She still felt devastated, so she began to eat ice cream, too. By now, her addiction to sugar was in full swing. Eating "over the top" of the feelings of her rage and betrayal only momentarily dulled the emotional pain she was feeling. By the time Janet entered therapy; she was eating large amounts of sugar at every meal and snacking on donuts in between meals. Her physical and emotional health was deteriorating rapidly.

When we are not in touch with our bodies and emotions, our relationship to food becomes similar to an unhealthy love affair. We are excited to be merged with our dysfunctional lover (lots of sugar and fat-laden food); but afterward, we are swamped with guilt and self-loathing.

When you are addicted to sugar, the first part of the process of learning to listen to your body's requests for food can be confusing. Many clients have said that when they checked in with their bodies about what they wanted to eat, they got this message: "You need to eat two bags of cookies!" That was their addiction talking, not their natural bodies.

In order to hear the true voice of your body, you may have to stop ingesting the offending substance until your body chemistry is balanced. So the first step is to gradually eliminate refined carbohydrates (i.e., sugar, white flour, white rice, white pasta, white bread and buns—in general, any white carbohydrate food) from your diet.

All refined carbohydrates can be considered addictive, but refined sugar is especially so. Because we have a tendency to underestimate the power of the cravings we have for sugar, it's best to gradually reduce your use of sugar. If you find that you just can't control your appetite for sugar, however, you may have to eliminate it from your diet entirely, at least for a while. Be patient with your process and allow your body to rebalance itself. As time goes by without your ingesting sugar, listen and notice how much better you feel. The more you crave it, the more you have been addicted. If you can stay the course you will begin to feel better every day. While you may miss the taste, you will enjoy recapturing your energy and your ability to concentrate. It's a good trade-off! And then one day you will find yourself craving a salad or green vegetables instead. That's a sign that your addiction to sugar is fading away. As that happens, you can begin the process of listening daily to your body's wisdom and trusting it to direct you in choosing your foods.

Once you are not "using" sugar as a drug, you may eventually be able to eat it in moderation with protein.

Many people who have experienced addictive behaviors say that their compulsive food habit is the most difficult addiction they've had to confront. If you have beaten other addictions (such as smoking, drinking, or drugs), you know how to be successful. Unlike other addictions, however, food is not a substance you can just stop ingesting. The road to recovery includes confronting your addictions at least three times a day—at breakfast, lunch, and dinner.

When you consistently eat junk foods, which "comfort" foods tend to be, you rob your body of the nutrition it needs, and poor nutrition sends your body a signal to increase body fat. Learning to respond appropriately to what your body requires and eating healthy foods that you enjoy can be among the most important experiences of your life. Eating can be a guilt-free pleasure that nurtures your body and your soul. The step-by-step plan described in Part II of this book will help you get to that place.

Overcoming the Addiction to Food

How do you know when you're addicted to something? You know you're addicted when you can't stop your behavior, even with the best of intentions, promises to yourself, and commitments to others. An addiction goes beyond willpower or just saying no. An addiction to food is a physical, emotional, and spiritual craving that demands relief through eating. Two common types of food addiction are bulimia and anorexia. Bulimia is an addiction to bingeing on food and then inducing vomiting and/or using laxatives to purge the food from the system. Just the opposite is anorexia, which is an addiction to not eating. As mentioned earlier, these eating patterns tend to first show up in adolescence or early adulthood.

The first tendency in facing an addiction is to deny it. In order get past this, look back through your life and be rigorously honest about your eating habits and any battles you may have had with food over the years. Whether you eat too much, not enough, or both, make some notes. Ask yourself how much of your time you spend thinking about, buying, and eating food. Do you think about food obsessively? It's normal to like food, but as a teenager or adult, it should be just *one of many things* you enjoy. If food is your greatest preoccupation or if you consistently overeat or under eat, it's important to look more deeply into your behavior.

The next step in any recovery program is to acknowledge the truth that you are an addict. Look at your habits. Do you overeat, make yourself vomit, take laxatives frequently, exercise obsessively, or under eat? All these behaviors are symptoms that your eating habits are out of control.

Overeaters Anonymous, Inc., is an excellent group to turn to if you can't control your eating habits. This program is confidential and is modeled on the principles of Alcoholics Anonymous, and it acknowledges food as the addictive substance instead of alcohol. This program supports individuals in winning their battle with food and helps people become normal eaters. Weight Watchers® is also an excellent organization that has helped thousands of people. Both organizations offer support in group settings. Overeaters Anonymous focuses more on the spiritual aspect of feeling out of control with food, whereas Weight Watchers focuses on portion control and emotional education.

The key is the sooner you begin the journey, the sooner you will be at peace with your body and with food. I know it is possible, because both of us have successfully faced our issues with food. If we can do it, so can you!

Cravings

Cravings are different from addictions. A craving is the compelling desire for one or two particular kinds of foods or perhaps an entire meal cooked in a certain way. You may think you are hungry, but you are not. True hunger comes on slowly. Your stomach rumbles and growls, then you realize you need to eat. With true hunger, you don't have the urge to eat any particular food, whereas a craving is an *emotional* demand to satisfy a hidden need by eating a specific food. So it's not really food you want. Look at the *feelings* beneath the craving for that special food.

John's story illustrates how cravings work. After working hard during the week, he would reward himself by ordering pizza for dinner. Every Friday night, he lounged in front of his TV, downed a few beers, and ate a whole pizza. As a result, he began putting on weight. Eventually, he decided to change his eating habits. He began working with Kathleen to improve his nutrition and with Linda to uncover his emotional connections with food. After some counseling, he decided to eliminate beer and large quantities of refined carbohydrates from his diet. That also meant cutting out pizza.

Everything was fine until John had a particularly hard week at work. An important contract was being negotiated and the office environment was tense. After lunch each day that week, John began craving pizza. When he finally closed the important deal, all he could think about was the taste and texture of his old favorite Friday night food. On the way home, it seemed that every restaurant he passed was a pizza parlor!

If John had not been prepared for this experience, he probably would have gone home, ordered pizza, and broken the agreement he'd made with himself. But Kathleen and Linda had told him to expect cravings and to know that there was an important feeling underneath them. As a result, he was willing to try some new behavior, even though he was skeptical. John had been taught that when he felt a craving coming on, he should sit still for ten minutes and do nothing about it. So John went home and sat on his couch in silence. He felt anxious and annoyed just sitting there, and he had to stifle a strong impulse to turn on the TV or "do" something.

Just before the ten minutes were up, John became aware that he was sad. Instead of avoiding his sadness, he allowed himself to feel it, and then to express it. He surprised himself by crying! As the tears ran down his cheeks, he realized what had been particularly hard about his workweek. John's personality was to be the "nice guy." He seldom raised his voice, and he disliked conflict. During that tense week, his supervisor had repeatedly yelled at him in front of other workers. John had felt ashamed and embarrassed. Although he'd acted as though his supervisor's behavior hadn't bothered him, he'd been deeply hurt by being treated that way.

When John finished crying, he felt so angry that he sat down at his computer and wrote a scathing letter to his supervisor. He even found himself yelling out loud as he wrote it! When the letter was finished, he printed it out, deleted it from his computer, and then tore the letter into a blizzard of small pieces. As John took a slow, deep breath of relief, he realized that his craving for pizza had disappeared. With a flash of self-awareness, John saw that all his adult life he had used food, especially pizza and beer, to suppress his pain and anger. It was easy to be a nice guy when he didn't let himself feel his anger. Part of John's recovery from his craving was to recognize *when* he was angry and to learn how to release that energy appropriately instead of eating "over the top" of his feelings.

Overcoming Cravings

If you are struggling with cravings, it's an excellent idea to keep a journal. Write down the thoughts and feelings you had just before the craving started. Because John was keeping a "craving journal," he was more receptive to his emotions when they surfaced. John had tried many diets in the past, but he had never been able to avoid his favorite foods when he had strong cravings. Each time he gave into them, he felt like a failure. He was tired of living the same old pattern and was determined to do whatever it took to break his habits. He became willing to cry and to express his anger.

Unexpressed feelings manifest themselves in a variety of behaviors. One of these behaviors is compulsively thinking about food. Another is being unable to control your impulses. To comfort yourself for feeling abused or victimized, for example, you may indulge in the impulse to eat sugary and/or fatty foods.

Some cravings are inherited. For example, people who have alcoholic parents are likely to be addicted to refined sugar and/or carbohydrates, even if they may not be addicted to alcohol themselves. (Later in this book, we will explain the relationship between the body, alcohol, and refined carbohydrates.) If the adult child of an alcoholic wants to overcome the craving for sugar, he or she will need to address the underlying feelings that lead to these cravings.

Expressing Our Feelings

As mentioned earlier, feelings are made up of energy. In an ideal world, we would express our feelings when they come up, or at least soon thereafter. If we don't, we store the energy of these feelings in our bodies. To overcome the habit of repressing feelings, we need to look at and process our feelings of vulnerability, victimization, sorrow, fear, pain, and anger. If the energy of these unexpressed feelings is not released, we can easily become ill.

As adults, we tend to act as though we are always strong. No matter how "put together" we are, we still have a vulnerable side. Guilt, insecurity, jealousy, fear, shyness, and sadness are examples of vulnerable feelings. Hidden vulnerability can haunt us. Always being the responsible or strong one is a heavy burden. Eating is one way to comfort those unconscious vulnerable feelings. Our vulnerability needs protection, and one way we protect ourselves from feelings of insecurity is through extra pounds. Many people habitually overeat, but don't ask themselves why. Acknowledging and feeling your vulnerable self and learning how to express anger appropriately are two major ways to break this cycle.

We have seen how our habits of eating stem from our earliest experiences with food and from the emotional patterns established in our families. Although this awareness is powerful, keep in mind that recognizing your feelings and permanently changing your behavior are only parts of a process. Advertisers love to tell you it's easy. Just buy their diet product and three weeks later your body and your life will be magically and effortlessly transformed! You'll be full of energy! If only it were that simple.

The goal of this book is to give you information and tools you need so that you can make peace with your body and enjoy your life without worrying about every bite of food you eat or how you look in a swimsuit. We want you to use your energy for experiences that fulfill you and can profoundly change your life. Seeing the "right number" on the scale can't give you permanent satisfaction. There is a way, however, and we will show you step-by-step how to achieve what you really want. Having a *Full Heart/Satisfied Belly* is not about being satiated with food. It's about being filled with life, energy, satisfaction, and enthusiasm. In order to connect with those positive feelings about life and our bodies we must take our power back from media images.

2

Debunking the Media Myth

If we are to believe all the advertisers, we must be slim and beautiful in order to be accepted, loved, sexually desired, and financially successful. Take a look at magazine and television advertising, for instance. How many ads do you see for weight-loss programs, beauty products, food supplements, and vitamins? What body types are most often seen on sitcoms and soap operas? How many of the female models are pencil-thin and the male models muscled and buffed?

We are bombarded incessantly with these unhealthy and unrealistic images. More than ever, our young children are being persuaded by these messages to believe that they, too, must live up to these "ideals" if they are to be successful. If we are to become truly conscious about eating, we must challenge these deeply embedded stereotypes of how we are "supposed" to look.

When you consider how frequently we're subjected to these images, it is somewhat ironic that more Americans are overweight now than ever before. It is no paradox that both anorexia and bulimia are on the increase. Overeating and under eating can both be attempts to mask the pain that is felt when the idealized version of how you "should look" and the way your body does look don't match.

A cover story in *People* magazine (October 30, 2000) was titled "Dying to be Thin." This five-page article described many of the drastic methods American men and women are risking in order to be thin. The six people featured in the article had all died in that pursuit. They died because they believed they would feel differently about themselves if only they could look like the current American ideal body image. That is a dangerous illusion!

The place you live, breathe, and experience your life is from *inside yourself.* If you think you will feel better when others approve of how you look on the outside, you are basing your self-esteem on someone else's opinion of you. That is the basis of the grand myth foisted upon us by the advertisements and commercials. Why do they do that? Because it's extremely profitable. Billions of dollars are spent every year to entice you into believing that with very little effort on your part, you can become permanently slender and thus entitled to live "the good life." What happens to all the feelings that were motivating you to overeat in the first place? What happens to all your negative thinking about your body? What happens to your inherited biological traits that determine your body type and how your flesh is arranged on your body? What happens to all your defense mechanisms that were protecting you from your underlying fears of the opposite sex? What happens to your appetite for connections to your self and to others and to spirituality that the food was replacing? Do all of these just magically disappear?

The answer to that question, of course, is no; but slick advertising makes you think that looking beautiful or handsome will permanently make all of your life issues simply melt away. Happiness is represented as something easily attainable by a simple adjustment of your body. No wonder they are making so much money. Remember, if they're spending a billion dollars on advertising, it's only because consumers are buying multiple billions of dollars worth of their products!

A hundred years ago, the same concept was peddled by disreputable traveling salesmen and it was called snake oil, some magic elixir that was supposedly capable of curing everything from hangnails to hair loss to gout. Selling the "magic" ingredient—be it a pill, a diet drink, or snake oil—is not a new concept. Deep in every human psyche is the profound longing for simple and easy transformation, something that magically requires no work. Marketing executives know that and they slant their advertising messages and visuals right to the core of that human longing.

We as humans have always desired the instant cure. The difference now is that television, the Internet, newspapers, magazines, and billboards have a much more profound influence on the images in our eyes and in our minds than the means of communication in generations past. The implication is that if our bodies don't match the images we see in the media, then we simply don't measure up. And if our bodies don't at least approximate that of a super model, then we aren't even on the same playing field.

How many super models are there in the whole world? Ten maybe? That means that the rest of us, if we're not careful, feel flawed because we are not one of the ten out of the billions of people on the planet! When you look at it that way, it seems pretty crazy, doesn't it? Wanting to be admired for how you look, however, isn't merely a cerebral idea; it is much more emotional than that. To really stop the destructive habit of comparing yourself to others, you must take the time to examine your underlying beliefs and begin to learn why the magazines, billboards, movies, and television shows affect you the way they do.

Granted, it's not going to be easy. Giving up the belief that a magic pill or effortless diet will quickly and automatically change your appearance, eliminate all your pain and discomfort, make you instantly desirable, and remove your insecurity is very much like giving up your belief in Santa Claus. The difference is that you probably believed in Santa for only eight or nine years. The idea of the quick fix has been repeatedly and indelibly stamped on your subconscious since the day you were born!

One of the first steps of disconnecting from the media myth is to begin noticing how most of the people on the planet really look. More than 99.9% of the world's population don't look like movie stars or cover models. The next time you're out and about, make it a point to look at the faces and the bodies of the general public. This is the first step, because it breaks the hypnotic trance that advertising creates.

Were you born with what you consider to be the perfect face and the perfect body? No, you say? Then you have three choices: (1) you can decide that you have been given an inferior face and body and choose to forever feel hopeless and miserable about yourself; (2) you can spend the rest of your life trying to change the way you look by diets, exercise, plastic surgery, makeup, and clothes; or (3) you can change your thoughts, disconnect from the media myth, and celebrate who you truly are. We realize that number three is the hardest; but even if you go all out on number two, you will still have to come ultimately to number three. Remember, you live inside yourself. No matter what the outside world tells you, your viewpoint, attitude, beliefs about who you are, your "lovability," and your attractiveness are all maintained inside your own head and therefore how you feel about yourself.

At an early age, Sandy bought into the media myth of the perfect body and spent most of her waking energy focused on her desire to transform her appearance to meet that illusory image. Sandy had been a yo-yo dieter since she first gained a few pounds at age thirteen. Having been a tall, skinny child up to that point, she felt chubby when her hips and thighs began to fill out. Her mother was always on some kind of diet, so cutting back on calories to lose weight seemed to be a logical solution to Sandy. Little did she know that she had started a behavior that would plague her for the next twenty years of her life.

When Sandy first came to see Linda as a client, she reported that after her first diet at thirteen, she lost weight. Within six months, however, she had regained that weight plus a few pounds more. The next diet was immediately begun and once again, she lost quickly, only to eventually gain it back with a few extra pounds besides. This became the pattern of her life. By the time she came to see Linda, she considered herself to be thirty pounds overweight despite having been on one diet or another for nearly her entire adult life! The only positive feelings she'd had about the way she looked over the years were the few months immediately after losing weight and before putting it all back on. Even those times, however, were overshadowed by the fear and the expectation of impending failure once again.

What happened to Sandy? Why didn't the diets work as advertised? What was she doing wrong? Sandy was addicted to the myth of instant success and even though her weight loss was never permanent, she never stopped hoping and believing. When the diets didn't work, she blamed herself for her lack of willpower and self-control. It was a never-ending cycle of hope and failure. Sandy, after two decades of self-punishment, was ready to give up.

Linda began by asking Sandy what her ideal self-image was. In other words, when did she feel her body was the most attractive and what picture of herself was she holding in her mind to compare herself to now? At first, she said she had no idea. After a few minutes of discussion, she realized that her ideal self-image when she was only thirteen, before she'd begun to develop physically.

Do something for yourself right now. Put this book down and close your eyes. Review how you have felt about your body over the years and see when you felt the best about the way you looked. Notice how old you were at the time and make a note to yourself of that age.

If your ideal body image was just a few years ago, that's to your advantage. If, however, it was when you were considerably younger (as it was in Sandy's case), you need to update your subconscious picture of yourself. Sandy was now thirty-three years old and upset with herself because she didn't look like she did at thirteen! Until then, Sandy had never thought about that tremendous age gap. She agreed it was both impossible and undesirable for a woman in her thirties to look like she had when she was thirteen.

As we continued to investigate this issue, Sandy updated her personal body image to a look appropriate for someone her age and discovered it was a much more reasonable expectation and only fifteen pounds different than her current weight! It took Sandy a few months of replaying her new self-image before she could entirely release that "ideal" of her body at thirteen years of age and finally let it disappear. She has since come to learn that one of the reasons people continue to be upset with themselves for not looking so much younger is because so many of the "adult" female models used in advertisements are actually underdeveloped teenagers!

The first step for you—as it was for Sandy—may be to come to grips with the fact that you have grown up and will never again be a teenager, or twenty or thirty or whatever age you have been holding in your mind. There are only a few people in the whole world who seem never to age. If you are one of those, be grateful. If, however, you are not, the first thing you need to do is to quit beating yourself up for having gotten older. No matter how you fight it, growing older is a reality and it doesn't have to be painful!

After Sandy had updated her self-image, we addressed the issue of the media image she was using as an ideal with which to compare herself. She was almost ashamed to admit that it was also a much younger female—Britney Spears!

Stop and think a minute about who possesses your ideal body image. Without realizing it, that visual may also be subconsciously reminding you of how you don't measure up physically. I challenge you to choose a more appropriate person to hold as your ideal. That doesn't mean you don't admire other attractive people and the way they perform. It just means you can forgive yourself for not looking like them. In Sandy's case, she chose for her ideal external model a thirty-year-old actress who played a lawyer on a television show.

Who would be an appropriate person for you to model your body style after?

Next, Sandy needed to address the habit she had of comparing herself to everyone else (and most of the time finding herself on the short end of the stick). During that period of her self-growth, Sandy was amazed to discover how often she noticed others who were thinner and more attractive than she thought she was. Rarely did she ever notice anyone whom she felt was her physical equal or not as attractive as she was. Instead, she automatically gave all her power and attention to those she considered superior to herself. It was not uncommon for her to become upset and leave a social gathering because she felt she didn't measure up physically to the others who were there.

This habit of constantly comparing ourselves to others has practically become a national pastime. In fact, it is such an ingrained habit in many people that they don't even know they're doing it. Once this habit is revealed, however, it can be healed. This is precisely what Sandy did. She gave up reading fashion magazines and watching television shows that featured all the actresses with whom she had been negatively comparing herself. By doing that, she took conscious control of the images she chose to embrace.

We began to focus on Sandy's physical positives—her eyes, her face, and all of her body's assets. It took her a few weeks to actually acknowledge that there were areas of her body that weren't so bad. Sandy had barely noticed that she indeed had a strong, well-proportioned body. She was hardly ever sick, she could walk several miles a day without tiring, and she was an excellent swimmer.

As Sandy began to appreciate herself more and more, she made another major discovery. She learned that she could control her thinking! She found that her thoughts were her own and that she could choose what she thought about. She had heard others talk about being able to do that, but she'd never actually practiced it before. That was the indication that Sandy was ready for the next step in her healing process: making peace with her body.

Whenever you are angry with your body for how it looks, for being sick, for how it is acting or feeling, you are at war with yourself. You would never put up with someone walking beside you twenty-four hours a day telling you how bad you looked or how poorly you were performing. Yet we too often do precisely that to ourselves. Learning to stop the negative chatter inside your head is an essential aspect of making peace with your body. Otherwise, no matter how well you look or feel, you will never be satisfied. Just to prove that point, how many people do you know that you think are very attractive but who continually tell you how dissatisfied they are with themselves and the way they look?

When you are constantly on your own case, you are giving your body all the wrong messages. Once again, that may be an unconscious habit you've been practicing nearly all your life. It doesn't matter how long you've been doing it; it's time to stop. Sandy began the practice of catching herself in a negative thinking pattern and bringing herself back to neutral. For instance, she caught herself thinking no man would find her attractive at a party she was about to attend. She immediately stopped that thought and remembered that of all the couples she knew, not one of these people looked like a movie star. She had grabbed herself back from the projection of the media zone!

As Sandy began to like herself more, compare herself less, and end the war with her own body, she began to lighten up emotionally. She gave up on diets and followed Kathleen's general guidelines about eating. She ate when she was hungry. Her fear was that she would gain lots of weight, and she did gain two pounds at first. However, she squelched her fears and kept listening to her body about what it wanted, instead of relying blindly on her diet mentality. Her weight and emotions both stabilized. Slowly over time, she lost twelve pounds and began to like her body image. The more satisfied she was with herself, the more fun she was to be around. When she reclaimed her power from the media and entertainment industries, her authentic self shone.

That was five years ago. Sandy is now happily married to a great guy and has a two-year-old daughter. Sandy has given up her obsession with comparing herself to others and basing her self-esteem on how she looks. She has chosen peace over perfection. In other words, she has come down from the moon palace. In the next chapter, we will tell you what that means and show you how you can come down from your own moon palace.

3

Coming Down from the Moon Palace

The mass media paint for us in living color the picture of the perfect body, the clean house, the harmonious and supportive relationship, the perfect job, financial stability, and clean, well-behaved children. It's an animated fairy tale!

Real people don't look polished in the morning eating their cereal. Real children make messes. If you try to keep your house looking like a model home, you'll miss out on all the joy and beauty life has to offer. When it comes to living in the real world, illusions must be left behind or you will be constantly disappointed.

Now more than ever, we are bombarded by images and messages that mislead us into thinking about how we "should" look and how our lives "should" be. The advertisers want you to believe their illusions so you will continue to buy their clients' products. In order to live an authentic life, however, you must come down from the moon palace. What that means is that you must give up the childlike illusions of the so-called perfect life so you can deal effectively with your everyday existence, for that is truly the real life.

Remember when we mentioned that giving up believing in the quick fix is a little like no longer believing in Santa Claus? Coming down from the moon palace is similar. It is only when you let go of obsessively longing for things to be different that you can begin to find solutions to your current challenges. When you are constantly yearning for the future or forever lamenting your past, you are not living in (nor allowing yourself to enjoy) the present. It is only in the present that you can appreciate and feel your life as it is right now. Feeling gratitude for your life and your body as it is right now, is an important aspect of being connected to yourself and is an essential ingredient of making peace with your body.

When you live in the moon palace of unrealistic expectations, you are inside a bubble of fantasies without benefit of a reality check—a bubble that is in danger of bursting at any moment and leaving you devastated. Here are some examples of people's "moon palace" thinking regarding eating and body image:

- If I looked like a movie star, I would be happy.

- Even though people keep telling me I'm too thin, I think I look great.

- If I could stop the aging process, I would be happy.

- If I were just two inches taller, I wouldn't look so heavy.

- If I weren't sick, I could be happy.

- If I just didn't get so hungry all the time, it would be easy to look good.

- If my thighs were smaller, I would be happy.

- I'm afraid of fat and avoid it in any form.

- I can't be successful, because my nose is too big.

- If I overeat, I must exercise even more strenuously to redeem myself.

- If I eat anything I like, I get fat.

All these thoughts are ways in which people disconnect from themselves by being critical and denying themselves the simple pleasures and joys of life they deserve. In the list above, it's obvious that happiness is being deferred until something changes. To do that is only to punish yourself, and then you are even *more* disconnected from your body.

Stop and examine your own life at this moment. What is it that you're waiting for before you change your health or how you look? We challenge you to come down from your moon palace and begin today what you have been wanting, but waiting to do!

Anne is a good example of someone who stepped out of the quagmire of her longing and waiting and moved forward in her life, even though she was afraid. When Linda first met her, Anne defined herself by her problems. She was over six feet tall with large hands and feet. She had always felt self-conscious about her height and felt she was awkward. She had bouts of chronic diarrhea and was extremely shy. Her voice was so soft that one had to listen to her very carefully to hear what she was saying.

For the last ten years, Anne's job was entering data at a computer company. While it paid the bills, she was starving emotionally. She dreamed of feeling healthy, secure, and also of being self-employed. You see, Anne had a hidden talent that very few knew about. Anne loved to sew. In fact, she was an excellent seamstress, having learned to sew when she was a young woman. She spent most of her time at work entering data, sipping diet cola, and daydreaming about making beautiful garments. She came to see Linda because her work at the office had been going downhill. She'd been making more mistakes lately and knew she was in danger of being fired. As each day went by, she became increasingly afraid of losing her job.

When Linda heard that Anne loved to sew, she encouraged her to do that for a living. Anne responded by spending the next thirty minutes telling Linda all the reasons why she couldn't do that. She had no confidence, she wasn't attractive, she had no people skills—the list went on and on. Linda, however, refused to accept the negative portrait Anne was painting of herself. Instead, Linda planted a small seed of hope and introduced Anne to the concept that it was no accident that she was making mistakes at work. Her body was trying to tell her something. It was trying to let her know that if it weren't for the income, she wouldn't even want to be there. Anne was waiting for something to happen that would make things different. Meanwhile, she was taking no positive action at all to make anything change. She criticized herself constantly and therefore felt inadequate emotionally and physically. As Anne and Linda began the process of identifying her negative thinking patterns, she realized that her internal chatter was her biggest enemy, and not the way she looked nor her assumed lack of people skills.

As she started to feel some hope about her situation, Anne relaxed enough to improve how she performed the duties of her current job. After a few weeks and feeling more secure, she took the risk of investigating the seamstress job market. The more she found out, the more excited she became. Six months later, she was hired by a small, local company where she could do what she liked best—sew! The power of being able to make a living doing what she loved to do gave Anne a new lease on life!

But her story doesn't end there. Anne carefully observed how the owners ran their shop, for she had not forgotten her dream of being self-employed. Within a short time, Anne took another risk and opened her own seamstress business. She has continued to work with Linda off and on for three years now. Anne no longer sees her height or shyness as anything detrimental to that which she is as a person. And by the way, Anne's recurring intestinal problem was easily solved when she gave up drinking diet cola.

Very seldom is the way you look the reason you can't do something. Behind that perceived inability is fear. It is a lot easier to blame your physical appearance than to face and tackle your fear as Anne did.

Learning how to discover your negative thinking, to be aware of your actions, and to identify the feelings beneath your behavior is the three-step process Anne used to connect to her personal power and set herself free. You can, too! Here are these three steps broken down:

Step One—Discovery

You must be willing to look beneath the surface of your outer behavior. Just as it was in Anne's case, sometimes you will discover that a crisis is an internal cry for help, if only you will look a little deeper. Anne's negative thinking blocked her power to change her occupation and thus her life. The same is true for changing careers as it is for changing eating habits. When you are blind to the deeper reasons why you are eating when you're not really hungry (or not eating when you know you're hungry), no behavioral plan will have lasting impact on your eating habits or your weight. It's never just about food. It's about the underlying thoughts and feelings you are attempting to mediate with food. Coming down from the moon palace also means becoming consciously aware of your thinking which, in turn, is causing your behavior. This is the first important step in the process.

Here are some common thoughts used to justify overeating:

Eating my comfort food makes me feel better. When you are experiencing feelings you don't like (depression, guilt, anger, or disappointment, for example), the idea of eating something comforting may become an overwhelming desire. You are convinced that the food will take the feelings away. That belief is often buried so deeply within your subconscious that you don't even realize you're not physically hungry. We find ourselves eating out of fear, pain, sadness, anger, the need for relaxation, energy, and company, or to fill the void inside. Seldom do we eat just because we are hungry. When you are reluctant to experience your emotions, eating becomes the only way of comforting yourself. In Chapter Ten ("Real Satisfaction"), you will learn how to distinguish between emotional hunger and physical hunger. We will guide you through a way to eat that will allow you to enjoy your eating experience in an entirely new and completely satisfying way.

I can get away with eating because no one will know. No one is around and the food is there. A rebellious part of you feels the overwhelming temptation to eat for no other reason than because no one is watching. You won't have to pretend you aren't hungry. You can eat something you normally wouldn't and you can eat with your fingers if you want to because no one will know! This has nothing to do with food. What are you angry about? How have you been depriving yourself and for whom? How are you disconnected from yourself? These are some of the deeper questions you want to ask yourself when you find yourself knee-deep in rebellion.

I deserve it. You've had a hard day. You deserve something wonderful to eat, even if it isn't on your food plan. You finally accomplished that big task, now you deserve a brownie. You got the promotion (or whatever), let's eat to celebrate! Often your parents, who rewarded your good behavior with food, started this habit. Now that you are an adult, however, there are other options you might want to consider. Some suggestions are taking the time to play, calling a friend, taking a hot bath, meditating, dancing, or trying something new you have always wanted to do. You're right—you do deserve to be rewarded. Food, however, is just one of many options you might choose.

I already blew it anyway. This could be considered rationalization at its finest. You already blew it by starting out the day with a donut, so why not have pizza for lunch? You're already bad, so why not just continue? The barn door is open and you are out of the previous constraints of your food plan. Your adrenaline is pumping and you have an irresistible urge to keep eating everything you have labeled as "bad." This sabotages the plans of even the most committed individuals. Even so-called "friends" will help you with your rationalization: "Just go ahead and eat it, honey...tomorrow is another day." Psychologically, once permission is given, the suppressed appetite is firmly in the driver's seat.

Since I won't get a chance to eat later, I must eat in advance, even if I'm not really hungry. This moon palace thinking is also used for feeling like it is the last time you will ever have an opportunity to taste those special chocolate cookies your Aunt Julie makes. They're so good, maybe you should have several more. Since you know you won't be able to eat lunch today, you eat twice your normal amount of food in a misguided attempt to avoid being hungry later.

Step Two—Be Aware of Your Actions

Objectively observe yourself. Have you ever eaten a whole package of cookies or candy or popcorn and weren't even aware of what you were doing? When you are diligent in observing your behavior, you can begin to do something about it. You still might overeat, but at least you know what you are doing, because it's impossible to stop unaware behavior!

Step Three—Identify the Feelings Beneath the Desire to Eat

Your feelings are really running the show. For instance, you may crave sugar when you are feeling overwhelmed. Feeling afraid might inspire a desire for pretzels and beer. Think about it for a few moments. What feelings do you associate with certain foods? How could you express those feelings instead of smothering them with food?

Ultimately, the goal of conscious eating is to receive the messages from your body about feelings and about food and to act on them. Being a conscious eater means giving yourself just the food you need and want and in just the right amount at the right time. To learn how to do that, let's start with the first step and examine the important role that denial plays in your life.

4

Dancing with Denial

According to the dictionary, "denial" is a rejection, the refusal to admit a truth or reality. In therapeutic terms, denial means not letting yourself know an underlying truth—usually about your feelings. For instance, instead of telling your friend that you're insulted by her comments about your life, it's quicker and safer to eat pizza or ice cream to bury your wounded feelings. To do that occasionally is not unusual. However, eating frequently to avoid feeling fearful, angry, sad, guilty, or any other emotion becomes a habit of denial.

Denial is a defense mechanism that keeps you from knowing an underlying truth that might create unpleasant feelings. Denial also keeps you from having to do something when you are not prepared to take action.

Harold is in a marriage where he is very unfulfilled. He and his wife share very little in common and have had no sexual intimacy for the last two years. On some level, Harold knows he should confront his dissatisfaction; but because of a variety of deeper feelings, he is afraid. To ameliorate those scary feelings, Harold unconsciously eats to excess. Countless failed diets and exercise programs have had no effect whatsoever on his extra pounds. His weight is an expanding energy layer protecting his vulnerable feelings. Until Harold is willing to confront the denial of his feelings about his marriage, his health and maybe even his life will remain at risk.

Realize that any activity you consistently overdo (work, think, exercise, play, smoke, talk, date, have sex, drink, take drugs, watch TV, work, play on the computer, spend money, or eat) is an attempt *not* to feel something. When you honestly admit what it is that you overdo, you can then begin to look for the unexpressed feeling that the activity is suppressing.

Denial also effectively blocks positive self-esteem, especially if you don't allow yourself to try new activities or learn new skills that could make you feel more competent. Your voice of denial may say, "You might get hurt or look foolish or embarrass yourself, if you do that! What if you fail? What will people say? Don't even try! You know you can't do it, so don't even put yourself in that position!" All these statements of denial are your defense mechanism misguidedly trying to keep you safe. These types of statements may have been true when you were a small child who didn't know the ways of the world, but now that you are grown, it's time to challenge such statements that are designed to keep you from stretching yourself and living a life of freedom and having peace of mind. The following are two examples of how denial can act as a defense mechanism.

Susan

Susan was contentedly focused on her work until her supervisor told her that she had made a critical error that would affect the whole department. "I can't believe I did that!" she exclaims. "I'll correct this immediately!" Her supervisor walks off with a parting shot, "Watch out, Susan. This is the second time this year one of your mistakes has held up the whole department!"

Susan's hand automatically starts searching for her stash of chocolate hidden away in her desk drawer. No time for lunch today! Not even a sandwich delivered from the deli. This is an emergency! She pops some candy into her month and immediately enjoys the sweet, reassuring, comforting taste. More handfuls of chocolate hardly register except when she has to wipe her hands to keep from getting chocolate on the computer keyboard.

After working several hours overtime, she's exhausted, but finally her error is corrected. Meanwhile, she has eaten her entire supply of chocolate. Her body is exhausted and she feels irritable. At the end of the day, Susan drives through the take-out lane at a fast-food restaurant and gets a hamburger, large fries, and a shake, and eats them in the car while driving home. *So much for my commitment to eat better quality food,* she thinks as she stuffs the last of the fries into her mouth. Later that night, she falls into an exhausted sleep and wakes up the next day cranky and feeling tired. She is resistant to getting up, let alone going back to work. In one sense, denial has served Susan by reducing the full force of her feelings about her mistake at work, including the fear that she could lose her job. The chocolate and fast food were unconscious attempts to feel better and push the unpleasant feelings away.

Better than drugs or alcohol, you might say. Yes, food is better than mind-altering drugs. But sugar and fat are in fact physically addictive substances. And just like all addictive substances, food is a short-term solution to long-term problems. Unconscious eating—justified because it was an "emergency"—kept Susan from adequately feeling and thus successfully processing her emotions about her error at work and her fear about losing her job. Does Susan's behavior sound at all familiar to you?

Most of us eat for emotional reasons from time to time. The difference between occasional emotional eating and a food addiction has to do with how often you indulge in the rationalization that food will actually help you cope with a situation. When you are in denial, you can't objectively observe yourself, because the denial blocks your viewpoint.

Linda's Own Personal Experience

"Food played only a small part of this event, but it serves as a good example of what can happen when significant feelings are not allowed to be experienced and expressed. When I was a young woman of twenty-two, there were complications that arose with my pregnancy. As a result, the fetus died in my womb and unfortunately nature did not take its course. I carried that dead baby in my womb for eight weeks! In the process of the eventual forced birth, I nearly bled to death. My mother cried, my husband cried, my whole family cried. During this whole experience, however, I never cried. My whole focus was to survive for my two little girls at home. In my attempt to be brave, I failed to shed a tear.

"Seventeen years later, I was at the gym in an aerobics class. Suddenly, I became extremely emotional. I was about to burst into tears and had not the slightest idea why. I abruptly left the class and drove straight home as fast as I dared. As I walked through the front door of my house, I had an intense desire to eat something. I curbed that impulse and made myself sit in a chair. Without warning, the memory of losing my unborn child overwhelmed me. The emotional pain that had been held trapped in my body for all those years surged through me in massive waves as I sobbed and sobbed. I mourned for the loss of my tiny baby for the rest of that day.

"Unexpressed emotions stay in your body until they are released. When you eat instead of appropriately expressing your feelings, the energy of those feelings remains trapped inside of you. In therapy, we call this 'eating over' the emotions. Susan ate over her fear and inadequacy. Likewise, my first instinct in feeling my old pain was to eat instead of cry. When you go through the process of losing weight, you may actually feel the old emotions that were buried under the extra pounds. It is important to express what the body has been holding, as I did when I finally mourned for my lost baby many years later.

"Denial does serve a useful purpose. As an automatic defense mechanism, it is the first stage of grieving in a time of acute emotional pain. Psychologically, it blocks the immediate feelings of emotional pain. Intellectually, the individual knows what has happened, just as I knew about the death of my baby, and Susan knew about her mistake at work. The intense impact of feelings is simply delayed for the moment. Denial is not something that is to be completely eliminated. In the illustration of losing my infant, my body and mind needed denial to shelter me from the acute emotional pain of that loss. The initial intention of denial is to be protective. In its natural form, denied feelings may last a few days or even a month or two before the painful emotions surface."

A Habit of Denial

When you have a pattern of denial, you are unable or unwilling to look at the deeper meaning behind your thoughts and actions. As a result, you remain frozen in your emotional development. This is common knowledge in the treatment of substance abuse, but is not so often recognized when food is the addiction. Here are some common ways denial shows up related to food and weight:

Lying—Many people lie to themselves and others about what and how much they eat, and they lie about how much they weigh. Anytime you exaggerate, minimize, or hide what you eat or don't eat, you are in denial. Addiction lives in the darkness. It thrives in secrecy. To break out of that pattern, start by telling the truth to someone you trust, someone who won't be critical of you. Begin the practice of eating in front of others. Allow light to shine upon your behavior and your feelings.

Ignoring Nutrition—Another common way of staying in denial is to resist nutritional information. I often hear people lament that there are so many experts contradicting themselves that they don't believe any of them. It's true that there are hundreds of approaches to the "right" way to eat and that every magazine has the latest new fad diet. However, not choosing to acknowledge what is known and proven and not taking responsibility for what works in your body is another way of staying in denial. It's also true that what works for one person will not always work for another. Still, there are some basics on which you can build a food program. These will be discussed later in Part II.

No Time to Think About It—One of the most common denials we hear is, "I don't have time to even think about what I eat!" Experiencing life at a constantly fast pace is simply "hurried sickness". Many people tell me they don't have time to assess what they want and need, let alone focus on a strategy to create it. When you are in that much of a hurry, it is easy to understand how you can become unaware of your own body's needs and why you might substitute quick food for relaxation and temporary emotional well-being.

When demands creep in through every crevice in your schedule, exhaustion is often the only feeling left at the end of the day. If there is no space for yourself in your life or if you don't feel any sense of accomplishment from a task, food might seem to give you the sweet taste of success you are seeking. If you feel like you are in that much of a hurry, it is time to slow down at least long enough to take a good look at how you are leading your life. It is time to reevaluate your priorities. Even if you are as busy as a single parent of eight children, you need energy and brainpower in order to be effective. That energy and brainpower comes from food. Are you so focused on everyone else's needs that you don't take the time to eat appropriately? The more stressed you are and the faster pace at which you run, the more important the quality of the food you eat becomes. The denial in this instance is buried in being over-committed to others and to tasks. Eventually, you will begin to feel resentful because your own basic needs are not being met. When that happens, your denial will make it seem as though it is someone's fault other than your own.

If the above paragraph describes you, it's time for you to be rigorously honest with yourself. Something has to give and, if you are not careful, it will be your health. If you are overextended, it's time to start saying "no" to everything other than those things that are absolutely vital. If you think everything is vital, you may need to consult a friend or a therapist to help you sort out your priorities. What *is* vital is your health. Your health depends upon you feeding your body and, especially when you are in stress, you need the best quality food you can find.

It's really not that hard to feed yourself well. As Linda recalls, "When I finally realized that I, too, was leading a rushed life, I purposely altered my eating habits by skipping the fast food and grabbing fresh produce, nuts, and whole grain bread instead. I even timed it. If I went through the express checkout lane at the grocery store, it didn't take any longer than using the drive-through at a fast food restaurant."

So what are your personal thoughts about eating, food, and time that might be indications of denial? Here is an exercise to help you examine them more closely.

1. On a piece of paper, list all your beliefs about food, your personal time, and about eating. The thoughts might make sense or not. In fact, they may appear to contradict one another. It doesn't matter. Just write them down without any self-judgment.

2. Once your list is complete, read each one carefully and answer the following questions: Is it really true? Have I been in denial? Does the thought serve me in a positive way? Or should I just reject that thought altogether? One of the benefits of this exercise is actually downloading all of your thoughts about this subject at one time. Many of your thoughts are so habitual that you may have never really seen them on paper before.

3. Once you have come face-to-face with your beliefs about these subjects, you can begin to monitor your thoughts consciously. Until now, those thoughts largely unconscious and, unbeknownst to you, have been running your behavior. Now that you have identified them, you can begin the process of changing the ones you determine should be changed. So choose the ones you want to keep, those you want to release, and those you want to change.

Here are some actual examples Linda has heard from clients and the choices they made about those thoughts:

- "I don't know how I gain weight! (I want to change this one—what am I ignoring?)"

- "I don't have time to prepare food in advance! It has to be quick or not at all! (I want to change this one—my time feels out of control.)"

- "When I am sad, candy makes me feel better. (I want to change this one—what is it that I am not feeling?)"

- "The best way to diet is not to eat anything I really like. (I want to release this one—I can't possibly be successful on any food plan I hate.)"

- "If I eat one cookie, I will eat the whole package. (I want to release this one—I am in charge, not the cookies.)"

- "All I have to do is walk by a brownie and I gain weight! (I want to release this one—this one keeps me feeling guilty for just looking!)"

- "I enjoy eating healthy foods like fruits and vegetables. (I want to keep this one—this is a healthy attitude!)"

Being aware of what we eat and why we eat are important parts of becoming conscious about the role food plays in our lives. Eating is often related to our unconscious emotional states. Many times, we cannot face the feelings, so we deny them and "eat over" them or stop eating altogether in order to avoid them. When we truly become aware of our habits, we have taken the first step toward changing them. We are then on the road to conscious and healthy eating. In the next chapter, you will learn how to focus on the practice of consciously listening to your body's needs.

5

Your Body Is Your Teacher

Your body is exquisitely designed to send you messages whenever it has needs that must be met. When was the last time your stomach growled, letting you know that your body needed food? Did you honor that sensation by feeding yourself as soon as possible? That was a simple example of your body communicating with your mind. Feelings of hunger, pain, discomfort, excitement, and joy are all ways in which our bodies communicate with our mental and emotional selves. Under the best circumstances, the body, mind, and spirit communicate as a well-organized team to create vitality, pleasure, and peace of mind. Ideally, you also act upon any warnings signs your body sends you.

Unfortunately, many people either don't recognize or they ignore the fact that physical messages are important. When we fail to heed these subtle messages, we can ultimately harm ourselves. Hunger, for instance, is a simple message from the body. The message of pain could be a muscle hurting from a new exercise program, or it could be an acute pain in your chest. If you have a habit of ignoring muscle pain, you might ignore chest pains, thinking it is indigestion. Many people have died because they didn't want to acknowledge the seriousness of the message of pain.

Because your body communicates with you by exhibiting a variety of symptoms, it is important to learn through the way you feel the specific language your body is using to speak to you. A few examples of the ways our bodies communicate with us are: headaches, apathy, back pain, neck pain, indigestion, painful and embarrassing gas, sleep disturbance, trembling hands, and mood swings. Exhaustion is another important example of the body communicating. If the message for rest is continually ignored, physical breakdown begins and ultimately illness or disease ensues.

Why is it that we don't instinctively act on the messages we receive from our bodies? There are a variety of reasons why we ignore the messages from our physical selves. Coming down from the moon palace means you have to take an honest look at your everyday behavior and your underlying emotional motivation. That process of discovery allows you the opportunity to get to the bottom of mindless eating. Honestly observing and recording your eating behavior on a regular basis is the first step in gathering the information you will ultimately need to change your behavior. (To help you with this process, see Kathleen's food journal in Chapter Fourteen.)

During her twenty years of working with hundreds of people on these issues, Linda has observed two major reasons people don't pay attention to body signals: (1) the "busy syndrome" and (2) "giving away our authority."

The Busy Syndrome

People are so busy "doing" that they often can't hear the quiet voice of their body. When you are overly busy, your mind is already focused on the next task to be done. Your eyes are on the future, not on the present. Lost in thoughts, you can be unaware of your body and the messages it is sending you. For instance, you might not realize something as basic as needing to go the bathroom. Or you could overlook the warning signs of an impending headache. Perhaps you ignore hunger signals or eat mindlessly. Linda says, "People who are so busy that they ignore the needs of their body, remind me of a cartoon figure I once saw with a huge head and big mouth, but with a tiny body. Such an image should remind us how easily we can diminish our bodies in this fast-paced mental world." Another of her clients, Linda says, was a perfect example of that caricature.

Eileen, a single, attractive, vibrant thirty-nine-year-old woman was a successful marketing executive who worked ten hours a day, six days a week. On Sundays, she sang in her church choir and then went to visit her mother in the nursing home. Eileen was always on the go. She seldom took any "down time" and when she did; she talked on the phone or watched television. She didn't think she had time to cook, so she ate fast food and highly processed items she could pop in the microwave.

When Eileen's body first sent her the message to rest, it was a gentle reminder. She began waking up in the morning still feeling tired. As she repeatedly ignored that message and drank more caffeine to stay awake, the reminders became more urgent. Eileen began to have trouble concentrating at work because she was so tired. One afternoon, she almost fell asleep at the wheel of her car while driving home.

Other symptoms then began to appear that were harder to ignore. She came down with the flu and even though she took a few days off work, she couldn't shake the symptoms. Then a sinus infection appeared. Eileen was so far behind in her work by this time that she didn't feel like she could stop again. Physical and emotional alarms went off saying, "Stop! Rest! Don't rush around! You need time to repair yourself!" Eileen persisted in overriding these messages, choosing instead to work faster and harder in a desperate attempt not to feel the fear that was building in her body. She was worried about her growing fatigue, lack of resistance to disease, and the mounting backlog at work. In an effort to feel some pleasure in the midst of all this emotional chaos, she doubled her intake of comfort food.

"I don't have time to stop now! There are deadlines to meet. I'll rest later," she told her body. But "later" didn't come. For almost a year, she ignored her body's messages. Finally, her body broke down and demanded the rest she'd been denying herself. She experienced a prolonged period of illness and was eventually diagnosed with fibromyalgia, an illness whose primary symptoms include muscle pain and chronic fatigability.

As have so many others, Eileen had ignored repeated prompting to rest because she keeps telling herself there were more important things that needed to be done.

You need to learn to trust your body, because it is an excellent barometer of your well-being. Each body is unique in the way it processes and communicates internal information. Therefore, learning to read your body's personal messages of hunger, feelings, sensations, satisfaction, and pain are essential to your health. It's impossible; however, to hear what is being communicated if you fill every moment of your life with activity or other distractions. When you are constantly racing against time, even if you are vaguely aware of your body's sensations, there is no energy to listen to them.

In therapy, Eileen slowly came down from the moon palace and began the first step by recording her food and daily activities in a journal. She started to notice that the more hurried she was, the worse she ate. She was surprised—and not just a little chagrined—to see the pattern of certain foods she ate when she was in stress. She was even able to rank her comfort foods as they related to her stressful feelings:

Lightly Uncomfortable	=	Popcorn with Lots of Butter
Considerably Uncomfortable	=	Ice Cream
Downright Stressed Out	=	Mexican Food
Beyond Stressed Out	=	Big Margaritas & Mexican Food
Out of Control (Crisis)	=	Wine & Italian Food

After Eileen had gone through the process of discovering what she was eating and how her stress and eating were connected, she was much more aware of her emotions and behavior. Awareness, as you will see in Part II of this book, as vital as it is to change, is only the beginning. How many of you are fully cognizant of what you are doing, but yet still do it? The next part of this process—identification—is where real changes are ultimately linked to underlying emotions and where old patterns can be broken.

Eileen discovered that the emotional issue that drove her to overachieve beyond that which was necessary or even healthy was her deepseated fear of not being good enough. In an elaborate attempt to overcompensate for her hidden and exaggerated feelings of incompetence, her immune system and subsequently her health were adversely affected.

Without healing the buried emotional reasons that drove her behavior, it was not possible for Eileen to end this destructive pattern. Over time and with direction and effort, however, she was able to release her beliefs of not being good enough and came to realistically accept her strengths and weaknesses. She learned to play and laugh again, and she learned to recognize her physical hunger and to eat high quality food. Eventually, Eileen was able to relax on a regular basis, learning to comfort herself with healthful activities. Through meditation, she was able to hear and honor her body's messages. She slowly mended her immune system and began living a more reasonable and satisfying life.

Eileen's experience is an extreme example of what can happen when one ignores physical symptoms. Unfortunately, not paying attention to what our bodies are saying to us is becoming more common every day in our society. Forgetting oneself usually begins in a small way. Take Matt and Fred, for example. These two men occasionally ignored their physical cues when it came to their jobs.

Matt often got so involved in his work that he forgot to eat lunch and then overate when he finally did stop long enough for a break. He has now learned to keep almonds and fresh fruit at his desk so he doesn't starve himself when he thinks he's too busy to go out to lunch.

Fred owns a construction business and gets up before sunrise. He says he is never hungry in the morning and so seldom eats breakfast.

Sometimes, he also forgets to eat lunch. Initially, Fred was really resistant to carrying food in his car. It took many months during which he was continually exhausted at the end of the day before he was willing to carry a cooler with such nutritious foods as fruits and vegetables. Fred has now learned to eat a little all day long and, as a result, he reports that he feels more energetic than he's ever felt before.

Your body is your vehicle. If you think you are too busy to fill your gas tank, how far do you think your car will go?

Giving Away Our Authority

The second reason for disregarding the messages our bodies give us is that we value someone else's ideas more than our own. Both Pam and Cindy were out of touch with their hunger.

Pam was twenty years old and living by herself for the first time. She ate three large meals a day plus snacks. Since this pattern of eating had been established early in her childhood, Pam believed unquestioningly that this was the way she was supposed to eat. It never occurred to her to check with her body to see if she was actually hungry. She assumed she was hungry simply because it was mealtime. Pam was also a "good girl" and cleaned her plate at every meal. In the process, she unconsciously overfed her body. When she came to see Linda, she had no idea why she continued to gain so much weight.

Cindy, a beautiful young girl of sixteen, read all the fashion magazines. She was out of touch with her body's hunger signs, because she ate so little. After reading the articles about models and the latest styles, she was convinced that she had to be super thin to be attractive to boys. In fact, Cindy was terrified of becoming fat. Between her extremely low intake of food and her intense desire to look like a model, Cindy was slowly—and literally—starving herself to death. She actually felt proud of never feeling hungry; in fact, she felt guilty when she did. Her body had begun to close down some of her basic processes in order to survive.

To everyone else, Cindy looked emaciated. In her own eyes, however, she was fat. Her whole sense of reality was distorted by the time she dropped to her record low weight of eighty-nine pounds. It was at that point that her mother took her to the doctor. The doctor, of course, immediately saw all the classic symptoms that the tests he later administered soon verified. Cindy was anorexic. She was in denial of one of her most basic physical needs, the need to provide her body with fuel in order to sustain her life.

While Pam and Cindy are at opposite ends of the spectrum regarding food and eating, both had conceded the authority to determine what their bodies needed to someone or something outside themselves. Pam was gliding through life on automatic pilot based on her parents' beliefs and habits about food. She needed to learn about nutrition and healthy eating habits and decide what was best *for her.*

What seemed right for your parents may not be right for you. In order to discover what is good for you, listen to your own body. Honestly observe how you feel and how your body processes the food you eat. Your energy level and overall health and well-being are clues your body uses to let you know what it needs.

In Cindy's case, she had adopted the image of a super-thin model as her authority. In the early stages of her eating disorder, whenever she was hungry, she would ask herself, "What would a cover model eat?" She based her dietary choices on what she thought her idol would do, rather than what was best for her. That was harmless enough at the beginning. However, it took a dangerous twist when her body began to fail her. When body fat is no longer available to burn as energy, the body begins to burn the tissues of the internal organs for fuel. At that point, the body is in crisis and it is absolutely critical that you immediately begin feeding your body highly nutritious food.

Anorexia is a complicated physical and emotional disease. Just wanting to look like a super model doesn't automatically create anorexia. Consistently denying and disconnecting from your own physical hunger, however, can establish a pattern that ultimately erodes your ability to recognize and respond to your natural hunger signals.

Linda reports that many times her body has let her know in absolute terms what it needed that she had been ignoring. "Once, I suspended my exercise program while I was recovering from a back injury. One day, I received a message from my body that said, 'Move me!' That wasn't a casual request, it was a demand! The message was so clear I immediately responded to it." That day, Linda began walking at least twenty minutes every day and hired a personal trainer. "By honoring a clear internal message," she says, "I strengthened my relationship with my physical self."

In another food-related instance, Linda says that she loved to start the morning with a hot cup of coffee, although she knew that she needed to eliminate caffeine from her diet. She says, "I started drinking decaffeinated coffee instead and then one day in meditation, I heard my body-voice say to me, 'Don't drink any kind of coffee again, not even decaffeinated!' This was also an urgent message, not at all subtle. Again, I followed the clear message and cut out all coffee from my diet. Eighteen months later, I was diagnosed with a bladder condition. The doctor told me I would have to permanently eliminate some things from my diet, one of which was coffee. I was pleased to report that I didn't drink coffee. What I didn't tell the urologist was that my body had already given me that important information several months prior to his recommendation!"

So how do you learn to listen to your body? The first thing is to slow down and honor any pain or discomfort you might have. Some people's mantra is "No Pain, No Gain." If you are an overachiever type, you may think that you either have to wallow in your pain or become a sissy. That's not at all what we're suggesting. What we're saying is that you need to stop denying your pain and learn to be gentle with yourself, when that's what your body is requesting. Many people push so hard on an exercise program that they seldom allow any deviation from their rigid schedule.

Honoring yourself means that if you wake up one morning and you are too tired to get up, you should listen to what your body is saying, instead of listening to what you think you *should* do. (On the other hand, if you have a tendency to resist exercise, you might think that your body *never wants* to get up and move!) Unless you are physically restricted—either temporarily or permanently—your body craves movement. Honoring your body doesn't mean letting your resistance to movement hold you back. It's up to you to be honest with yourself as to which side of the fence you tend to be on. Are you inclined toward too much exercise or too little? The best plan, of course, is somewhere in between. Here are some simple ways to begin to improve your communication with your body:

1. Learn to distinguish between emotional and physical hunger. Eat only when you are physically hungry, and develop nurturing ways of meeting your emotional needs without food.

2. When you are tired, stop and rest for a few moments, take a few deep breaths. When possible, take a nap. Avoid drinking caffeine to override fatigue and using drugs and/or alcohol to induce relaxation.

3. If you are always too busy, make it a point to free up a few hours of empty time to literally do nothing. Does that suggestion scare you? Be honest about your resistance. Do you say you would like to do that, but still never create space for yourself?

4. Begin a regular practice of being quiet and sitting in that stillness. If you have never done that before, begin with five minutes and gradually increase that time to twenty minutes or more.

5. After you have become comfortable sitting in silence, learn how to meditate. You will find an exercise to guide you through that experience in Part II of this book.

6. Get a massage. Don't talk or go to sleep during the massage. Concentrate on where your body is being touched and gratefully receive that sensation.

7. Pay attention to your body's aches and pains. On the other hand, don't overreact and imagine the worst. Allow your pain to be an indicator, a message that your body is trying to tell you something. Try accessing that message from the body by keeping a journal, meditating, visualizing, or just being open to that information whenever and from wherever it is presented to you. You could even be in a restaurant and overhear a conversation that gives you your answer. The key is to remain open and receptive. Of course, you should always seek a physician's advice if you're experiencing acute or persistent pain.

8. Resist the temptation to overdo physical exercise. A personal trainer once told Linda that the most common mistake people make in exercise training is that they exercise too much. Your body needs time to rest between periods of physical exercise.

In addition to the small voice of your body that speaks to you, there are other methods of communication your body can use that are just as effective in relaying physical information. Some people can literally hear their bodies talking to them, while others communicate visually. While reading a book about health, an answer about your body may leap out at you. Or perhaps you will sense that you need to eliminate a certain food from your diet without knowing exactly why. If you are more kinesthetic, you may best communicate with your body during physical activity. In other words, there is neither a wrong way nor one right way in which to receive information. It is important and affirming to give yourself credit every time you receive guidance. Act on it, and see if you experience a benefit. If you don't, make a note of that fact, too, and continue to practice improving your communication with your body. By choosing to read this chapter, you have already begun! And in the next, you will begin to learn how everything—and everyone—is connected to one another.

6

Our Connection to the Earth

We all seek to understand the most basic of relationships, as somewhere deep within us is the reality that all of us are indeed connected to one another, to the earth, to ourselves, and to the source of life. This innate awareness helps us see how the links in the chain of food production—from seed to the soil, to fertilizers and pesticides, to harvesting and packaging—are also all interrelated. When we put food in our mouths, we become a part of that chain. For at least a couple of generations, we have been separated from knowledge of this food chain by the commercialized, processed, grocery store presentation of our food. We have lost sight of the fact that we are one with everything we eat and how what we eat affects us and our vitality, our very life force.

Traditional cultures that live close to the earth have always known that we are not separate from nature and our food. Indeed, we are one organism, as Chief Seattle, of the Suquamish Indians in the Pacific Northwest, stated well over a hundred years ago:

> *We are part of the earth and it is part of us. The perfumed flowers are our sisters. The deer, the horse, the eagle, these are our brothers. The rocky crests, the juices of the meadows, the body heat of the pony and man—all belong to the same family. For whatever happens to the beasts soon happens to man. All things are connected. This we know. The earth does not belong to man. Man belongs to the earth. This we know. All things are*

connected. Whatever befalls the earth befalls the sons of earth. Man did not weave the web of life; he is merely a strand in it. Whatever he does to the web, he does to himself.

This section is intended to make you more aware of how food in the United States is grown and produced. We will look closely at the differences between commercially produced and organically grown foods. As you become more conscious about how food is grown, you can make healthier choices about what you serve yourself and your family. Simple choices, such as what you eat each day, can have a positive impact on your health and on the well-being of our planet.

Commercial farming has changed significantly in the last fifty years. Much of the food in the American diet today is unhealthy. Before World War II, however, agricultural practices were safer for people, plants, animals, soil, and water. What happened?

The Use of Pesticides

Chemical pesticide use in the United States has grown over 3000% since 1945, creating a significant impact on our health and the health of those who grow our food. Farmers who are in constant contact with pesticides have seen their risk for getting cancer rise to six times that of the rest of the population. In addition, thousands of farm workers are poisoned or become permanently sterile each year, according to *Your Guide to Organic Power: Positive Choice for the Earth and You* (Wild Oats Markets, Inc., 1998). As a professional nutritionist, Kathleen is keenly aware of the impact pesticides have had on the health of many of the people who come to see her.

Recently, one of her clients, a principal in a nearby country school, was complaining of chronic fatigue. When Kathleen asked her if there were any toxins in her environment, the principal said that as far as she knew, she had not been exposed to chemicals either at work or at home. When Kathleen questioned her a little further, she learned that her client's school was located next to a large farm. "Check with the farmer to find out what he sprays his crops with," Kathleen advised, "and ask him what time of day he does his spraying." A week later, she gave Kathleen the answer. The farmer had told her that he sprayed his crops with pesticides during school hours.

Hearing this, Kathleen sent the principal to an environmental specialist to have her tested. The test results revealed that her body was on toxic overload. Chemicals sprayed on the nearby crops showed up in large quantities in her body and her physician felt this contributed significantly to her chronic fatigue symptoms. Kathleen's client was instrumental in getting the spraying stopped during school hours. Her actions undoubtedly helped prevent further harm to herself and to the other teachers and children, even though the location of farm next to the school still posed a potential health hazard.

Ironically, insects that were supposed to be eliminated by pesticides have become resistant to the chemicals being used on them. To combat this situation, increasingly potent pesticides have been developed and greater amounts are being sprayed on crops. A Environmental Protection Agency (EPA) report released in the mid-1990s stated that each year an estimated 911 million pounds of synthetic pesticides are applied to conventional agricultural crops in the United States. The EPA considers 60% of all herbicides, 90% of all fungicides, and 30% of all insecticides to be potentially cancer causing.

The EPA also has found ninety-eight pesticides in our groundwater (including DDT, which is a banned substance) in at least thirty-eight states. One alarming statistic points to the harm these pesticides have created: tests done in Michigan in 1976 found PBBs (polybrominated biphenyls) in mothers' milk. In his book, *Diet for a New America,* John Robbins says that this chemical is a known carcinogenic substance and can cross the placental barrier and cause physical defects to the fetus. The women were unaware that through their breast milk they were passing PBBs to their infants.

Chemical Fertilizers and Soil Erosion

In addition to the health hazards caused by pesticides, our soil is also threatened. We are losing three billion tons of topsoil each year, a rate seven times faster than nature can rebuild it. This is due in part to the fact that the soil is becoming so depleted by the chemicals used to fertilize it and the chemicals sprayed on the plants growing in it that it is being rendered sterile, bereft of the microorganisms necessary to break down organic matter (corn stalks, for example) that revitalize the soil. Further, there is not enough vegetation or trees on the commercial farms to anchor and protect the soil or to stabilize the water table when it rains. As a result, the soil lies barren and exposed to the elements of wind and rain, which wash it away.

Vernon Carter and Tom Dale in their book *Topsoil and Civilization* point out that wherever soil erosion has destroyed the fertility base on which civilizations have been built, these civilizations have perished. World history is replete with wars that were fought over land that was needed to feed the people. As a country became more prosperous, one of the signs of wealth was the abundance of food on the tables of its citizens. To maintain this lifestyle in the face of a growing population, it was often necessary to seize agricultural land from neighboring countries. Conflicts from territorial disputes would become more frequent until the people of the other countries rebelled and toppled these ancient empires, whose greed and mismanagement of resources contributed to their demise. Will history repeat itself once again?

As the soil becomes thinner, greater amounts of chemical fertilizers are used to increase food production. This is a short-term solution with long-term ramifications. These fertilizers destroy beneficial microorganisms, worms, and insects. A vicious cycle is created—the depleted soil requires increased chemical fertilizers, which in turn cause weak plants, which are easy targets for insects and diseases, which then require higher use of pesticides, fungicides and herbicides. In a variety of ways, these chemicals end up in our water and air supply, in our food, and in our bodies.

The Science of Seeds and Food

Genetically engineered food (sometimes referred to as a genetically modified organism, or GMO), is a new, corporation-driven form of food. Companies are hiring scientists to take genes, the very building blocks of life, and manipulate them in order to change the nature of plants. By cutting, splicing, and transferring genes between totally unrelated living things, they have succeeded in producing combinations that do not occur naturally. They are also introducing genes into plants mostly using viruses, purportedly to produce stronger, healthier plants. More than forty varieties of crops have already been genetically engineered (including at least half of our soybeans, half of our cotton, and a fourth of our corn)—in total, more than two-thirds of the foods on the shelves of your local grocery store.

Unwittingly and certainly without our permission, we have each become a human experiment. There are no regulations requiring companies to inform consumers that their food products have been genetically engineered or altered. Unless it is clearly marked that a particular food product does *not* contain GMO, it most likely does.

Another problem with genetically engineered plants is that they do not produce seeds capable of replicating themselves. As a result, farmers have no choice but to purchase all of the genetically engineered seeds from the corporations that manufactured them in the first place. And most farmers, quite frankly, are blind to what concoction they are actually planting.

This is a new area in which we are playing with fire and there is no one on duty to extinguish the flames. It is, therefore, up to us as consumers to be aware and not buy these foods.

Follow the Money to Learn What Keeps This Poisonous System Going

Crop rotation is a simple way to reduce the need for pesticides and fertilizers, but farmers who do this don't qualify for government-funded crop support programs. In addition, many banks that lend money to farmers and the companies that insure them require farmers to use pesticides.

Another reason that drives this harmful system is that pesticides are big business, particularly in the United States. Our country is one of the world's largest users of pesticides, herbicides, fungicides, and seeds that have been genetically engineered and altered. Sales for pesticides alone are close to eight billion dollars a year in the United States. In addition, American companies export more than *twenty-five tons of pesticides an hour* to other countries. Many of these pesticides we're exporting are banned from use in the United States! Foreign farmers use these pesticides and then sell their crops back to us. The result is that pesticides banned in the United States continue to be present in many of the foods we buy, particularly fresh fruits and vegetables.

Commercial Production and Animals

Animals raised for food consumption pose an even larger problem to our health than crops, because animals eat the plants that have been treated with all the chemicals discussed above. More than 95% of all the toxic chemicals in America's diet comes from meat, poultry, fish, dairy products, and eggs. In particular, cows, pigs, and poultry are fed large quantities of artificial hormones, growth stimulants, pesticides, insecticides, tranquilizers, radioactive isotopes, chemical colorants, and antibiotics. When we eat the meat from these animals, we take into our bodies the chemicals contained in theirs.

Antibiotics

You will perhaps be amazed as we were to learn that more than half of all antibiotics manufactured in the United States are given to animals or put into animal feed. Granted, antibiotics kill harmful bacteria. Over time, however, the bacteria adapt to the antibiotics, so that the drugs are no longer effective. Newer and stronger antibiotics are then developed to kill the same bacteria. The European Economic Community has banned American meat that is infused with antibiotics because the organization strongly believes that these chemicals are unhealthy. In contrast, our pharmaceutical and meat industries and many of our politicians do not consider meat laced with antibiotics to be a problem. It is becoming increasingly apparent that the interests of big business seem to be more important than the interests of public health.

Hormones

Hormones in farm animals pose yet another health danger. Hormones are given to farm animals to increase milk and egg production and to develop heavier livestock for slaughter. Hormones are potent substances that are naturally secreted in minute amounts by the glands of all animals, including humans. These hormones control our entire endocrine and reproductive systems. Our bodies are sensitive to even minuscule amounts of hormones, yet we ingest large doses of artificial hormones through animal products daily.

Dr. John Monaco, author of *Slim and Fit Kids,* writes: "If bovine growth hormone makes cows gain weight, it doesn't take a great leap of imagination to assume it may have the same effect in our children." As disturbing as that is, weight gain is only one concern created by these hormones. Monaco says that some evidence suggests that hormones in food may be causing early puberty in children.

The Energy of Our Feedlots

The animals that most of us eat are raised in overcrowded, assembly-line conditions. As a result, these animals pass their saddened, angry spirits on to us in our food. Since all life is connected, we ingest not only the meat, but the feelings of the animals as well.

Do we want to be connected to this misery and anger?

As we have seen, we are paying a high price for commercially grown food—we take into our bodies harmful chemicals from plants and animals, our soils are depleted, and our health is at risk. Clearly, what happens to our plants and animals affects us directly. What can we do about these conditions? What are our options?

Positive Choices: Organic Foods

The answer is simple. We can buy organically grown foods, which are commonly available in health food stores (which are expanding throughout the United States) and in specialty sections of regular food chains. When we receive life essence from clean food, our bodies become more vibrant. Nutritious, healthy food helps us feel more vital and alive.

Organic fruits and vegetables are free of pesticides, herbicides, and fungicides. Many animals are also raised without hormones and antibiotics and are treated with respect. They are fed organic foods and live in natural habitats rather than in the crowded, unhealthy conditions in which nearly all of animals raised conventionally are forced to endure. "Free range" chickens, for example, are allowed to roam outdoors in the air and sun. They have fewer infections, stronger immune systems, and appear to be much more contented animals. This is in stark contrast to conventional chickens that are packed into crowded, dark spaces in which they are unable to move. Commonly, the beaks and claws of these chickens are forcibly and painfully removed so they cannot peck or scratch. Their natural behaviors are done away with. Considering all this, what is it that you are really eating?

The "Firman Bear Report" on research conducted at Rutgers University found that organic food was not only safer than conventionally grown food, but also that it contained greater concentrations of vitamins, minerals, and enzymes. The overall results of this research showed that the organic foods studied contained 87% more minerals and trace elements than food that was conventionally grown.

What is *Organic*?

We know that organic food is healthy, but how do we define what is and is not organic? In 1980, the United States Department of Agriculture (USDA) stated that organic farming is a production system which avoids the use of synthetically compounded fertilizers, pesticides, growth regulators, and livestock feed additives. According to the USDA, to the maximum extent possible, organic farm systems rely on crop rotation, crop residues, animal manure, legumes, green manure (plants that are left to replenish the soil), organic wastes, mechanical cultivation, mineral-bearing rocks, and biological pest control to maintain soil productivity, supply plant nutrients, and to control insects, weeds, and other pests.

"Organically grown" means more than the absence of pesticides, herbicides, and synthetic fertilizers. It is actually a different philosophy. To the organic farmer, soil is alive, teeming with millions of organisms, from bacteria to earthworms. It nourishes plants, animals, and human beings. Organic farmers treat the earth and its creatures with respect. You are eating food and animals that are filled with life and nourishment. And in doing so, you are receiving vitality and a positive life force through your food.

Organic Standards

As of October 21, 2002, any food sold as organic has met criteria set by the United States Department of Agriculture. It is called the USDA's National Organic Rule. The food is stamped with a green and white seal if it is produced without hormones, antibiotics, pesticides, herbicides, insecticides, synthetic fertilizers, or genetic modifications. The rule uses different terms to distinguish different levels of purity:

- 100% Organic: Products carrying this label cannot contain any non-organic ingredients.

- Organic: At least 95% of the product's ingredients must be organic.

- Made with Organic Ingredients: Must contain at least 70% organic ingredient. Should not contain any added sulfites.

- Some Organic Ingredients: Products containing less than 70% organic ingredients and can list them individually.

- Before this time the Organic Trade Association, an organization independent of both the farmers and the government, regulated the organic industry with rigid standards. Organic farmers are still required to observe these rules:

- The land must be free of prohibited chemicals for three years prior to organic certification

- The grower or processor must keep detailed records of organic methods and materials.

- All methods and materials are inspected and certified yearly by a third party.

When you are buying food be aware, however, of foods designated as *All Natural or Pesticide Free*. This does not give you adequate information to discern in what environment the food was grown. If you see a food marked *Transitional*, it tells you that the farmer is committed to changing a conventional farm to an organic one, but it takes at least three years to change the practices to organic.

What About Cost?

When people consider buying organic food, the question of price often comes up. It's true that organic sometimes costs more than conventionally grown products. (The price of organic food is steadily decreasing as more people demand them, so cost is quickly becoming less of a deterrent.) What we don't see in conventional products, though, are the hidden costs involved in their production. These costs include federal subsidies to farmers, pesticide regulation and testing, and hazardous waste removal and disposal. Also, our taxes are used to fund the $8 billion farm subsidies program. Other hidden costs are harder to put a price tag on. These include health problems (headaches, sleep disorders, digestive problems, cancer, infertility, for example), behavioral problems (violent outbursts, anxiety, depression, attention deficit disorders, etc.), and environmental damage that can result from the widespread use of unhealthy chemicals.

Of course, we can live healthier lives and save money by eating smaller amounts of food than we normally eat, thus offsetting some of the cost of organic food. More importantly, however, what price do you place on your health and vitality? What are you worth to yourself and your family and friends? Are you making food choices that are infusing you with a vital life force, or are you making choices that are depleting you?

Remember, we not only absorb the life force and vitality of food itself, but also the energy and state of mind of everyone who handles it—the workers in the seed companies, farmers, harvesters, truckers, grocery store employees, and those who do the shopping and cooking. We are all inextricably connected. Before we eat, we can take a moment to think of all these people. We can bless them and the food that will sustain our bodies. This practice makes us consciously aware that we are all connected and that everything we do has a ripple effect on everything (and everyone) else. It makes us grateful for the blessing that food is to us.

Marion

Another of Kathleen's clients is Marion who writes in her own words of the vital role that organic food has played in her life.

"On February 28, 1991, at age forty-five, my life took a sudden turn—on a journey I could never have imagined. I received from my doctor a report of surgical pathology about a lump I had found in my groin. The words on the report were all foreign. None of them really made sense to me. I struggled to understand what I was reading. Then the words in the diagnosis came looming out at me—lymph nodes, biopsy, malignant lymphoma. I was Stage Four of the disease. A very serious prognosis, I was told. I was advised that we needed to treat it aggressively.

"For the next six months, I had rounds of heavy doses of four chemotherapy drugs, after which I was told I'd gone into full remission. We celebrated! My husband threw a huge party celebrating my return to full health. We invited all our friends who so generously helped with their love, cards, and prayers. It was a fabulous party with at least fifty friends joining us in celebrating our relief of the cancer's remission.

"Ten months later, in a routine mammogram, they found enlarged lymph nodes under my left arm. The news that the cancer had returned was so much worse than the initial diagnosis. I was devastated. I was waiting to undergo a stem cell transplant and did more chemotherapy to prepare for it. I went into partial remission, so I was given the option to 'watch and wait' instead of moving forward with the transplant. I jumped at the idea. I played this watch-and-wait game for two years. Every three months, I went in for a checkup only to be told that although I was not sick enough to be treated, the cancer was still in my body. I was told it may get worse; but by then, there may be a cure. This game was one I was not enjoying.

"On Christmas 1995, my sister-in-law gave me a book she thought I'd enjoy. Little did she realize that it would change my life forever. *Spontaneous Healing* by Dr. Andrew Weil opened my consciousness to the fact that our bodies have the natural ability to heal themselves, if we only give them the tools they need and treat them with the dignity that they deserve.

"The book began my journey of holistic healing that I continue to practice today. My enlightenment with the help of a nutritionist and colon hydrotherapist brought me into full remission in two months. The symptoms that I had started to display went away in a month—like a droopy eye from a nerve that was being pressed on by an enlarged lymph node and several enlarged lymph nodes under my left arm.

"I learned that food is not just about pleasure, but that it also has a very important function—to nourish the body. I also learned that chemical-free organic food was critical to my liver and immune system so that they would have the ability to fight my disease. I continue to eat clean, healthy food. My life depends on it.

"The bottom line is that I learned to honor my body through my experience with cancer. The cancer took me to the realization that nutrition is the key to my health. My spiritual journey through food allowed me to embrace eating consciously, which means I no longer feel as if I am depriving myself to eat this way. I eat what I do out of love for my body and not from the fear that the cancer will come back. This seems minor, but it has been a journey out of fear to one of honor and love of myself."

It is true that you are what you eat. What you put in your mouth makes a difference because food strongly affects the quality of your life. If you want abundant energy and a clear mind, clean, healthy food is a must. Healthy, responsible eating helps enhance your vitality, strength, and well-being, and it helps raise your spiritual awareness. Further, your emotional state can become more balanced so that you can take charge in navigating your life instead of letting events control your life. The choices you make ripple out to other people, animals, plants, and the earth. What choices will you make?

7

How Our Body Works

Now that we've begun to understand how the production of food affects us, let's examine how we connect to ourselves. Because our lives are so busy, we aren't in the habit of listening to our own bodies. As a result, what your body needs and the signals it's sending you may go unnoticed.

This chapter will help you understand how your digestive system works. This knowledge will assist you in making more informed choices about what you eat. Because you are a complete and integrated system, what you do to one part affects the whole. As you're reading, think of the digestive system not as separate from the rest of you, but as an important and interrelated part of your whole being.

The Digestive System

Mouth

The digestive system starts with the mouth where our teeth break food down into small, easier to swallow pieces, with more surface areas for digestive enzymes to act on. The longer you chew, the better it is because you are giving the enzymes in your saliva more time to do their job. In fact, carbohydrates start their digestive process in the mouth. Your mother was right—take time to chew your food!

Esophagus

After swallowing, your food enters the esophagus, a muscular tube about twelve inches long. Its job is to transport food and liquid from the mouth to the stomach. When food enters the esophagus, its muscles start a wave-like, squeezing motion, called peristalsis, from top to bottom. This action moves food down to the stomach. At the boundary where the esophagus meets the stomach, well-developed, smooth muscles keep food from flowing backwards into the esophagus.

Once the food reaches the stomach, it is churned and covered with acid. The stomach lining can handle this acid, but the esophagus lining cannot. If you eat too much or too fast, you might feel a burning sensation in the chest area close to the heart (which is why it is commonly called "heartburn," although it's medically known as "acid or esophageal reflux"). This could indicate that there has been some passage—a reflux action—of the food back into the esophagus, which can cause pain and belching. People also refer to this as "indigestion" and often seek medical help to relieve it. This is another important reason to eat slowly and chew your food well!

Stomach

Cup your hands together. This is about the size of your stomach. The amount of food we normally eat is much larger than this, so the stomach has to stretch to accommodate it. Those "super-sized" portions we are encouraged to eat by fast-food chains, however, are far larger than the stomach is intended to handle. Think twice before indulging in them.

The stomach produces the enzymes and hydrochloric acid necessary for digestion, especially the digestion of proteins. Many people take over-the-counter antacids to relieve the pain of indigestion, but these stop the production of the very acid we need to break down protein. The best way to avoid reflux is to eat smaller amounts of food and to chew each bite thoroughly.

Food remains in the stomach from about thirty minutes to four hours or longer, depending on what was eaten and how much. Alcohol and water are absorbed directly into the blood from the stomach, but other foods continue on their digestive journey.

Small Intestine

The small intestine is about twenty-two to thirty feet long. The thick, soupy fluid—called chyme—that results from food being mixed and broken down in the stomach, moves to the first part of the small intestine, the duodenum, which is about ten to twelve inches long. The duodenum, which is connected to the pancreas and the gall bladder, plays a major role in digesting our food while the rest of the small intestine helps assimilate nutrients from our food. Juices released from the pancreas into the duodenum bring enzymes to aid digestion, along with enzymes produced in the small intestine itself.

The gallbladder releases bile, which has been made in the liver, into the duodenum to help digest fats. This process also neutralizes the acid from the stomach and creates an alkaline environment in the small intestine. This is very important because nutrients, which will be transported into the blood, must first be in an alkaline state similar to that of blood for this process to take place.

Chyme remains in the small intestine for about four to eight hours, depending on what was eaten and how much. The small intestine needs to be healthy, with strong peristalsis and good bacteria, to properly do its job of absorbing nutrients. Nutrients find their way into the blood and lymph system through small hair-like projections called villi, which must be unclogged and porous in order to be effective. If they are gummed up with the residue of refined foods, absorption is difficult. When you were a child, did you ever make paste with flour and water? This is what your white flour and sugar products break down to in your intestines. They create a paste-like substance that covers the villi. When the body can't absorb nutrients, it feels as if it is starving, no matter how much food it's getting.

The primary purpose of eating is to nourish the body. The body needs whole foods, not refined foods, to keep the digestive tract functioning. Although the effects of refined and other foods will be discussed later, we cannot stress enough how important it is to have a well-functioning digestive tract. When it does its job well, it contributes to our total well-being, which includes mental clarity and balanced emotions.

Large Intestine/Colon

At the end of the small intestine is a one-way valve (the ileocecal valve) that allows the chyme to pass into the large intestine. The large intestine—or colon—absorbs about one-fourth of the fluid from the chyme. It also absorbs electrolytes and forms solid waste. The colon is an important part of the digestive process and the healthier it is, the better it can do its job. The colon is about five to six feet long and has loose, bellows-like pockets called haustra which are muscular structures that facilitate the movement of waste material through the large intestine. Friendly colon bacteria manufacture vitamin K and some B vitamins along with some of the antibodies that are needed by the immune system.

There are many parts to the large intestine. The ileocecal valve empties chyme into the first and widest part of the intestine (about two-and-one-half to three inches in diameter) located on the right side called the cecum. The appendix is a finger-like projection off the cecum. The ascending colon is next. Chyme moves slowly uphill against gravity in this area and then makes a sharp turn as it approaches what is known as the hepatic flexure. If elimination is sluggish, the ascending colon can become very distended and congested.

From there, the chyme moves sideways into the transverse colon, the largest and most movable section of the colon. The transverse colon will sag from the weight of solid matter if it remains in the colon too long. In this area, water is removed from the chyme, which now becomes solid matter. If the body is dehydrated, it will take what water it needs from the waste, which can render the waste very hard and difficult to evacuate. The solid matter must now make its way past another turn (the splenic flexure), and then enter the descending colon on the left side of the body.

***

How Much Water Should You Drink?

Your body is made up of at least 70% water. The formula to determine the amount of water you need to drink each day is to divide your body weight in half. The result is the number of ounces of water you should drink every day. For example, if you weigh 150 pounds, you need to drink as a minimum 75 ounces of water (*i.e.*, 150/2 = 75).

***

Peristalsis keeps the solid matter moving into an area called the sigmoid. The sigmoid is shaped like an "S" to keep waste matter from emptying into the rectum too quickly. The rectum has an opening called the anus that has two sphincters (muscular rings) that help control the evacuation of stools. (Thank God for this design!)

It is very important to keep the colon clean and filled with the good bacteria that produce vitamins, stimulate the formation of antibodies (which protect our bodies against infection), remove toxins, and help eliminate gas.

The whole digestive process—the time it takes for food to pass through the whole tract and be eliminated as waste (transit time)—is approximately twenty-four hours. You can test your transit time by getting some frozen organic corn. Put a small handful in your mouth and swallow them whole with some water. Note the time and date they went in your body and then look for them to exit the body in your waste. The intervening time is known as your transit time.

This is a good time to mention that although it is sometimes necessary to take antibiotics, it's important to know that they indiscriminately destroy not only infectious bacteria, but beneficial bacterial flora as well. It is a good idea to replace these helpful bacteria when you are finished with a course of antibiotics. You can purchase a good probiotic (good bacteria of the bowel) from your local health food store. When you replace helpful bacteria, you restore good bowel health more quickly.

Liver

Other than the skin, the liver is the largest organ in the body. It is located in the upper right section of the abdomen. Because of the abundance of blood within the liver, it is a deep red color when healthy. The liver is an important chemical factory that controls diverse functions essential for maintaining life. One-fourth of the heart's output flows through the liver at all times.

The liver produces bile, which aids digestion. In addition, the liver extracts toxins from the body and breaks them down so the body can eliminate them. It synthesizes, dissolves, and stores amino acids (proteins) and fat. The liver also produces and stores glycogen, a substance that stores energy in order to regulate blood sugar levels, and it stores various vitamins in forms ready for use by the body. The liver also adjusts metabolites (substances critical to the metabolic process) that are circulating in the bloodstream. If all this weren't enough responsibility, the liver also regulates the volume of blood by storing it and releasing it as needed, it breaks down old red blood cells, it stores iron, and it helps in the production of antibodies (gamma globulin)!

The liver is obviously a powerhouse. It is vital to life, but especially to the *quality* of life. If your food lacks nutrients and is loaded with chemical residue, antibiotics, and hormones, your liver becomes overtaxed and congested. This is another reason why organic food is so important to your body. Alcohol, which is broken down by the liver, is actually a toxin to the body. If your liver is not functioning well, neither are you.

Pancreas

The pancreas weighs only a few ounces and is about six inches long and is located behind the stomach. As mentioned above, the pancreas produces digestive enzymes, but it also secretes insulin and glucagon, which regulate the amount of glucose in the blood. Insulin will be dis-

cussed a little later, but first we'll examine the importance of the digestive enzymes.

Digestive System

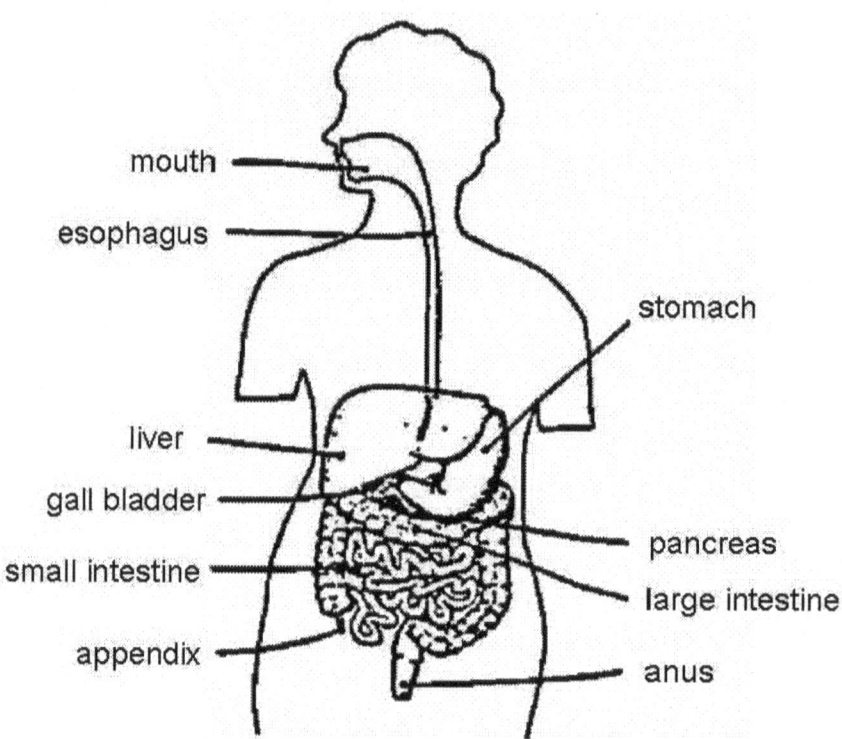

Enzymes

Life could not exist without enzymes. Enzymes digest our food so that
it becomes small enough to pass through the minute pores of the intestines into the blood. Enzymes in the blood take digested food and build
it into muscles, nerves, blood, and glands. They are responsible for a
healthy immune system, bloodstream, liver, kidney, spleen, and pancreas, as well as our ability to see, think, and breathe.

Enzymes act upon one substance and change it into a different substance, either a chemical or byproduct, while the enzymes themselves remain unchanged. A substance that an enzyme acts upon and changes is called a substrate. For example, the substrate might begin as protein in the form of a piece of chicken. Enzymes attach to this protein and change it to amino acids that go into the blood. Other enzymes and substances turn the amino acids into muscle.

There are three major types of enzymes: metabolic enzymes, digestive enzymes, and food enzymes. *Metabolic* enzymes are produced from the nutrients we eat. They work in the blood and in all organs and tissues. *Digestive* enzymes are made by the stomach, intestines, pancreas, and other organs and break down food. *Food* enzymes are found in foods, especially those that are raw. This includes all fruits and vegetables and sprouted foods when they are eaten uncooked.

Enzymes are destroyed at 129 degrees Fahrenheit and in other procedures used in the processing of food. Therefore, all canned, pasteurized, baked, roasted, stewed, and fried foods lack enzymes. Nature has placed enzymes in food to aid in the digestive process, instead of forcing the body's enzymes to do all the work. But when we eat cooked and processed foods, our digestive systems have to produce all the enzymes. This causes an enlargement of the digestive organs, especially the pancreas.

Eighty percent of your body's energy is used in digestion. If you are run-down, under stress, living in either a very hot or very cold climate, are pregnant or nursing, are a frequent air traveler, or eat a diet high in cooked, processed foods, your body requires enormous quantities of extra enzymes. In addition to the enzymes used in digestive fluids (including salivary and intestinal secretions), we also lose enzymes naturally through sweat, urine, and feces.

With our American diets relying too heavily upon processed foods, we are working our digestive systems to the maximum. Since our digestive systems cannot produce all the enzymes our bodies need, they are forced to draw on enzyme reserves from organs and tissues, resulting in a deficiency of metabolic enzymes. As a result, we don't feel energetic and our emotions are often less than positive. Worse than this, general malaise is the fact that a lack of enzymes can create an environment ripe for disease.

It's apparent, then, why it is so important to eat fruits and vegetables in their natural state. The easiest and best thing you can do to create a healthy digestive system is to eat plenty of green, leafy salads with mixed organic greens (not iceberg lettuce, however, because it has very little nutritional value and gums up the intestinal wall) and cut-up, raw vegetables and fruit. (This book does not cover sprouted foods, which also add enzymes to your system, but you can find books on this subject in local bookstores.) Canned and cooked foods, for the reasons discussed earlier, do not have much nutritional value. But if you eat something raw with each meal, you will bring life and vitality to your body, instead of draining it during the important digestive process.

Ask yourself where you think you'll be in the aging process ten, twenty, or thirty years from now if you continue to eat mostly cooked and processed foods and especially if you have any of the stresses listed above. Are the diseases and physical decline normally associated with aging actually due to growing older? Or are they due to our nutrient- and enzyme-deprived diet? We believe the latter is true.

Our bodies are designed to give us feedback. When a part of the body is in pain or discomfort, it is signaling us to listen and make changes. It is easier to learn the language of the body when we understand how it works. This chapter gave you an overview of the digestive process. If you'd like to learn even more, we suggest you enroll in a basic "Anatomy and Physiology" course at a community college. The wonder and awe you will experience from this knowledge will be invaluable.

Connectedness to our body is easier when we understand how it works. Understanding how different foods affect our connectedness to our bodies, emotions and mood is also helpful in this journey.

8

SAD: Our Standard American Diet

Many people, especially those with families, feel that they don't have time to shop for groceries, let alone cook. As a result, increasingly large numbers of Americans eat most of their meals away from home. Single people don't like to come home from work and eat all by themselves, so they also prefer to eat out. We have convinced ourselves that our lives are so busy that we can't take the time or make the effort to think about what we eat. Joan and Christopher provide us with good examples of this.

Last night after work, Joan went to a fast-food restaurant and ordered a super-sized cheeseburger, some french fries, and a diet cola. This morning, she ran out the door without eating breakfast. At work, she stopped at the vending machine and bought a shrink-wrapped Danish pastry and grabbed a cup of coffee from the office kitchen. After feeling the zing from the caffeine and sugar, she felt she was ready for her morning. At lunch, the manager sent out for pizza and diet cola for everyone in the office.

Because his wife goes to work before the rest of her family gets up, her husband Christopher is responsible for making breakfast every morning. He doesn't want the hassle of cooking anything, so he gives their children sugarcoated cereal with milk, a cola, and toast made with white bread and margarine.

As the family bolts for the door, Christopher gives the kids their lunch money. At the end of the day, his wife comes to the family's "rescue" by stopping for tacos and burritos on her way home from work.

Scenes such as these are played out day after day in homes and offices all across our country.

What are we *really* eating? How much nutrition is there in the foods we typically eat?

Fast foods and restaurant foods contain more fat, sodium, refined carbohydrates, additives, and chemicals such as monosodium glutamate (MSG) and aspartame, than food prepared at home. These foods from commercial eating establishments encourage overeating with their large portions and good taste. But they are loaded with fat and empty calories. They do not nourish us.

In this chapter, we will see how the most common foods in our American diet react in our bodies. Understanding the nature of food and its role in the body will help us see which foods keep us connected to our inner wisdom and which foods cause disconnection. We can use this information to help us make thoughtful food choices. We will concentrate on fats, carbohydrates, aspartame, and caffeine because they are so prevalent in our diet, which Jack Tips, in his book *The Weight Is Over,* aptly calls the Standard American Diet (SAD).

Fats

The subject of fats is confusing for all of us. For years, we have been hearing how "bad" fats are. Advertising urges us to buy "low-fat" and "fat-free" foods. Simply because cookies, for example, are advertised as low-fat or fat-free, we are duped into believing they are healthy. Since they are low in fat, we don't worry about gaining weight, and then proceed to eat four or five cookies at a time. What we don't realize is that it is the cookies' high sugar and salt content that actually causes weight gain. In fact, we need fat to be healthy. Our bodies require essential fatty acids; but since our bodies can't produce them, we must get them from food.

There are three essential fatty acids: *linoleum acid* (LA), also called Omega 6, found in nuts, seeds, whole grains, and dark green vegetables; *alpha-linolenic acid* (ALA), also called Omega 3, found in flaxseed oil, pumpkinseeds, walnuts, soy, and dark green vegetables; and *arachidonic acid* (AA), found in meat. (People in the United States usually have an excess of this acid because they eat a lot of animal products.)

Essential fatty acids are important because they:

- Promote healthy skin and hair
- Support proper thyroid and adrenal activity
- Bolster the immune system
- Are necessary for normal growth and energy
- Promote healthy blood, nerves, and arteries
- Are crucial in the transportation and breakdown of cholesterol
- Are essential for hormone production, especially prostaglandin, a hormone-like substance which controls cellular functions, lowers blood pressure, and inhibits blood fats from sticking together

Obviously, we need fats in our diet. In fact, our body should be about 20-25% fat, and we can develop health risks when our body fat gets much higher or lower than this. The greatest health risks are to the heart and blood vessels, which is why we have such a high rate of heart attacks and strokes in this country.

Kevin, for example, was overweight and had high cholesterol at the age of thirty-seven. Because Kevin was at risk of heart disease, his doctor sent him to Kathleen for nutritional counseling. Kevin had a desk job. His diet consisted mostly of fast foods. He found that they were convenient and besides, they tasted good. When he learned about fats and how they work in the body, however, he was willing to improve his diet. Kevin's father had died of a heart attack in his mid-fifties. Kevin did not want to repeat history.

The best food sources of essential fatty acids are:

- Raw nuts and seeds
- Whole grains
- Legumes
- Flaxseed oil
- Walnuts
- Soy products
- Dark green leafy vegetables
- Fish
- Oils from evening primrose
- Oils from black currant and borage seeds

Olive oil, safflower oil, almond oil, and flaxseed oil can be sprinkled on salads and steamed vegetables. They can also be mixed in blended drinks (commonly called "smoothies") that are made with fresh fruits and vegetables. You can use olive oil to sauté vegetables or to baste vegetables on the grill. Buy unrefined oils that have been mechanically pressed and oils that come in cans or dark glass containers. Be sure to store oils in a cool, dark place, as oils become rancid when they are heated or exposed to oxygen and light.

Fried Foods

Foods that are fried are placed in fat heated to 320 degrees Fahrenheit or higher, causing the original structure of the fat molecule to be altered, rendering it incapable of fitting properly into the body's cells, thus harming the integrity of the cell membrane. This means that the cells cannot absorb certain nutrients or keep harmful substances from entering or exiting them. The chemical structure formed by heat is called trans-poly-unsaturated fatty acids (TFA), more commonly known as trans-fatty acids. Trans-fatty acids interfere with the enzyme systems that metabolize natural fatty acids and can cause deficiencies of these necessary fats.

Simply stated, fried foods are dangerous for our bodies. <u>Fried foods deplete our bodies physically and provide our bodies with no nutritional value whatsoever.</u> It's important to avoid fried foods and solid fats like margarine and shortening and other products made with solid fats and hydrogenated or partially hydrogenated oil.

Want to know what fried foods do to your body? Buy some fried chicken, and leave it on the counter overnight in the original container. The next morning, look at the chicken and see the solid fat that has congealed on it. Smell the chicken. The solid fat and unpleasant smell will show you what your blood and other organs would be dealing with had you eaten the chicken. This type of fat sticks to your arteries and blocks them, making it difficult for nutrients to travel where they need to go.

Other factors that block essential fatty acids from being used in our bodies are:

- Alcohol and tobacco
- Radiation, including low-level radiation from electronic appliances (TVs, computers, cell phones, etc.)
- Aspirin and other synthetic drugs
- Free radical activity in the body, especially in excess
- Over-consumption of animal products
- Deficiencies of vital nutrients, especially vitamins B3, B6, C, E, zinc, and magnesium

Cholesterol

We're accustomed to thinking of cholesterol as the "bad" fat, but cholesterol is actually essential for life. In fact, it's not a fat, but a pearly white, waxy alcohol.

Cholesterol has many functions:

- Every cell in the body requires it to maintain the structural integrity of its membrane, to control the flow of water and nutrients into the cell, and to send waste products out.

- The nerves and brain require it for normal electrical signal transmission.

- The body uses cholesterol as a building block for many important hormones, especially the sex hormones and hydrocortisol, the body's natural steroid.

- Cholesterol in the bile of the liver aids in digesting fatty foods and helps absorb fat-soluble vitamins A, D, E, and K from food.

- Cholesterol gives the skin the ability to shed water.

Every cell in your body can make cholesterol, but most of it is made in the liver. When the supply of cholesterol in the cell is low, it either makes more cholesterol or sends messengers to the cell surface to collect some from the bloodstream. You will always have cholesterol in your blood, unless something is drastically wrong. Falling cholesterol levels are often a marker for cancer, which is one reason doctors check the blood for cholesterol levels.

Elevated blood cholesterol is often an indication that the diet is too high in cholesterol and saturated fats (usually animal products and fried food). Doctors also monitor low-density lipoprotein (LDL) and high-density lipoprotein (HDL). Since neither cholesterol (a waxy solid) nor triglycerides (the storage form of fat) are soluble in blood, the only way they can get around is to be wrapped up and carried by the lipoproteins that are soluble in blood. Lipoprotein acts as an envelope that encloses cholesterol and triglycerides so they can be transported to the tissues. LDL carries cholesterol from the food and liver to the cells. HDL takes unused cholesterol back to the liver to be processed and excreted, usually through the bowel.

Humbart Santillo, N.D., points out in his book *Intuitive Eating* that a high LDL indicates that the body is becoming overloaded with fats and doesn't have the proper nutrients to get rid of them. High HDL means that the body is getting rid of excess cholesterol and preventing it from accumulating. Neither one is bad (LDL) or good (HDL), in spite of what you hear. What is important is to look at the ratio between them. Health risks are monitored by this ratio.

The two benchmark standards* are:

- Total cholesterol divided by HDL should be below 4.0
- LDL divided by HDL should be below 3.1

* Note, however that benchmark standards may vary from lab to lab.

The positive thing about these ratios is that you are primarily in control of them. Again, it's about conscious choices. You can regulate healthy levels of cholesterol, LDL, and HDL by paying attention to the foods you eat.

Ann came to see Kathleen after being told by her doctor that she had high cholesterol and poor HDL/LDL ratios. She did not want to go on cholesterol-lowering medicine because she'd heard that it has some unwelcome side effects. She was a busy bank officer who ate a lot of fast foods and stayed alert by drinking coffee and diet cola. She also attended a number of business lunches, never thinking twice about what she selected from the menus. She didn't have a weight problem and so assumed she didn't have high cholesterol. Ann now wanted to learn all she could about those things that create high cholesterol levels. Kathleen told her about the harmful effects of eating a diet high in saturated fats, refined carbohydrates, and chemicals like aspartame, which is found in diet cola. When Ann realized what she was doing to her system, she immediately began choosing more nutritious foods.

With time, the new way of eating became Ann's normal, everyday way of eating. One year later, her cholesterol ratios were in the normal range, and there was no need for her to be on cholesterol-reducing medication. As a welcome bonus, she experienced more energy and greater mental clarity.

Fat and Weight Loss

Many of Kathleen's clients who come to see her in an attempt to lose weight have been on low-fat diets. They are pleasantly surprised when they are told to add healthy fat (in moderation, of course) to their diet. And what happens when they do? They start to lose weight and enjoy food again! You see, the body needs healthy fats and is genetically set up to desire them. Long ago, when we were hunters and gatherers, fats kept us alive during the lean times. If we deny ourselves fat in our diet, our bodies will work against us and our cravings for fats will become overwhelming. On the other hand, if we eat too much fat, our body will automatically store it. We simply need to make conscious and wise choices about what fats we eat and in what quantities.

Gail was experiencing horrible hot flashes and sleepless nights. Her doctor was unable to regulate her hormones. She was gaining weight on a low-fat, 2000-calories-a-day diet. She was understandably becoming discouraged, and she was about to give up. She came to see Kathleen who suggested she start adding three tablespoons of flaxseed oil and a supplement containing clean fish oil to her diet every day. At first, she was horrified at the idea. Fat had long since become the enemy! When Kathleen told her about the importance of fats and that she needed essential fatty acids in order to burn fats, she was willing to give it a try.

Within just a couple of months, she was sleeping at night. Importantly, her doctor was able to regulate her hormones, and that alone was a huge relief. The big bonus as far as Gail was concerned was that she started to burn fat. Not only that, her skin, hair, and nails took on a new luster and strength, and a lot of the cravings she used to have were gone.

Carbohydrates

Carbohydrates include all starches and sugars, such as fruits and vegetables, grains (such as bread, pastas, chips, cereals, rice), alcohol, (beer, wine, whiskey, etc.), potatoes, candy and desserts (for example, cakes, cookies, pies, pastries, donuts, ice cream), and regular sodas. Carbohydrates all break down into simple sugars which are easy for the body to burn; in fact, they burn cleaner than protein and fat. There are two basic types of carbohydrates: *simple* and *complex*. During the last 60 years, however, we have added a third type: *refined* carbohydrates.

Simple carbohydrates are found in fruit, many vegetables, and in milk. They require little digestion and enter the bloodstream quickly. Complex carbohydrates, found in vegetables and whole grains, require more of the digestive process and help control the conversion to glucose (sugar). Remember, glucose (sugar) is the body's energy fuel. Simple and complex carbohydrates also contain fiber, which does not convert to sugar. Fiber controls the rate at which sugar reaches the bloodstream.

Refined carbohydrates are found in a number of foods including refined white table sugar, refined flours used for fillers, pastries, pastas, rice cakes, white bread, cookies, cakes, desserts, and gravies. Instant mashed potatoes and most boxed cereals also contain refined sugar and grains. These foods deliver sugar to the body very quickly, which challenges our system, as we will see later. Refined sugars have low nutritional value. What little nutrition there is comes through chemicals added to replace nutrients lost in processing. Refined carbohydrates have had a negative impact on our health because we are not genetically set up to handle the refined products we have engineered. These foods are causing a rise in adult onset diabetes (also known as Type II diabetes), heart disease, strokes, hormone imbalances, some cancers, and mood disorders.

The November 1998 issue of the *Nutritional Action Newsletter* addressed sugar consumption in the United States: "The insatiable American sweet tooth has done it again. In 1996, the latest year for which figures are available, our intake of refined sugars rose...for the tenth year in a row. Enough sugar was produced to provide every man, woman, and child with 152 pounds of refined sweeteners, table sugar, high-fructose corn syrup, dextrose, etc. That's an overestimate, because all the sweeteners produced don't necessarily reach our mouths. But you can still use those figures to compare one year to another. And in 1996, we averaged twenty-five more pounds of sugar per person than we did in 1986."

Remember that these figures do not include refined flour and refined grain products. Our bodies are in trouble.

Sally came to see Kathleen because her three-year-old son David was out of control. He would have a tantrum whenever he didn't get his way. If Sally sent him to his room, he would throw things, cry, and scream until he was exhausted and fell asleep. He didn't have any friends and was expelled from his preschool because he screamed uncontrollably and hit other children. Sally had taken him to a doctor who concluded that nothing was physically wrong with her son. A friend suggested he might have allergies and need a change in his diet.

When Kathleen first saw her, Sally was confused and desperate. She wasn't a permissive parent and couldn't understand the extreme behavior her child was exhibiting. Kathleen went over David's diet and discovered that he was eating almost all refined carbohydrates and sugar. Cookies, candy, and cola kept him from throwing tantrums for short periods of time and, in fact, got Sally through the grocery store without being embarrassed. David ate donuts and sugared cereal when he refused the meals she fixed for him.

Kathleen sent David to a doctor who tested him for allergies and found that David was very allergic to milk. This was one of the "good" foods he would eat, so Sally had been giving him a lot of chocolate milk. Sally wanted a good relationship with her son, and she couldn't live with him the way he was, so she was willing to go through the process of withdrawing sugar from his diet. It took a little over a year to change his diet to nutrient-dense foods, but it was worth it. His behavior improved markedly as his body received what it needed.

Insulin

To understand how carbohydrates affect us, we need to look at insulin. Insulin is a powerful hormone that is poured into your blood when the pancreas gets the message that your blood contains sugar. Insulin binds with sugar and carries it to your cells. Insulin also acts as the key to unlock your cell walls so that sugar can enter the cell where, once inside, the sugar can be used for energy.

When insulin is turned on in excess, it functions in ways that do not support your health. For instance, excess insulin will increase the storage of fat. When there is too much sugar in the blood and cells don't need to burn it for energy, it is stored as fat. Insulin also regulates the body's production of cholesterol by directing the liver to make LDL to carry the fat, which is a consequence of eating refined carbohydrates. (High levels of LDL stick to blood vessel walls and form plaque, putting you at increased risk of heart disease and stroke. You may also feel dull and lifeless.)

Insulin also drives your kidneys to retain fluid. Excess fluid puts you at increased risk for hypertension and heart disease. In addition, insulin promotes smooth muscle growth in blood vessel walls which can cause rigidity, leaving the vessels vulnerable to plaque. All of this contributes to a breakdown of the vessel walls. Your blood is responsible for many things, including carrying oxygen and nutrients to cells and carrying waste away from them. If blood flow is slowed down as it passes through narrowed vessels, your whole cardiovascular system is compromised.

If your rings are tight and your socks leave an indentation around your ankles that takes hours to go away, try this experiment. For one week, eat a diet of two pieces of fruit, all the vegetables you want, (fresh or steamed), three to four ounces of protein at each meal, and drink eight to ten eight-ounce glasses of pure water a day. If you find yourself urinating a lot and the puffy feeling dissipating, you may be having an insulin reaction from refined carbohydrates in your diet. It's important that you check with your physician to determine the exact cause.

Refined Carbohydrates

Refined carbohydrates have a direct relationship to our moods. When you eat refined sugar, for example, your body moves the sugar from your blood and into your cells for storage. Refined carbohydrates don't allow the sugar to be released into the bloodstream slowly the way it should be, as there is no fiber in refined carbohydrates to buffer the sugar release. As a result, you experience an energy drop shortly after you eat refined sugar, a drop which comes from low blood sugar (hypoglycemia). This is the same reason why you often feel so tired an hour after a meal. Low blood sugar also causes restlessness, poor concentration and memory, frustration, irritability, and unexpected anger.

Sugar also has a direct connection to serotonin and beta-endorphin, chemicals in the brain which regulate self-esteem and well-being, increase stability and optimism, cause feelings of peace and relaxation, and help control impulsive behavior. Sugar acts in the brain much as these chemicals do. The problem is that over time, you need more and more sugar to get the same good feeling, and you soon find yourself addicted to sugar. You need it to feel good. At the same time, you also find it harder to cope with life. For instance, you may feel scattered and depressed, fly off the handle, feel tearful and overwhelmed, and crave sugar to the point where you are eating it uncontrollably. Add these symptoms to those from low blood sugar, and you can understand why you are having a bad day.

Another problem with refined carbohydrates is that they lack nutrients. When our nutrient level is low, a part of our brain picks up the message that we're starving. This primal part of our brain served our ancestors well. When food was scarce, it told the body to store fat for the lean times—fat that could be burned for energy as needed. Most of us don't have lean times now, because food is in abundant supply. Still, that part of our brain continues to pick up the signal that our body is starved, so we keep storing fat. Before long, we are overweight, tired, and ill.

A lot of people are addicted to refined carbohydrates. Kathleen admits to being one of them. "Most of my life," she explains, "I have craved bread, desserts, candy, and chocolate. As a child, my favorite treat was toasted white bread smeared with margarine, sugar, and cinnamon." As an adult, her more "sophisticated" tastes demanded rich desserts and chocolate. "If someone set a box of chocolates in front of me, I would sit there and eat and eat until they were gone," she admits. "Chocolates were gloriously satisfying as I ate them, but about half an hour later, I felt horrible. I was light-headed. In addition to being dizzy, I felt tired and couldn't think straight. I felt like I either needed more chocolate to pick me up or I needed a long nap."

Kathleen says that many of her clients are in the same boat as she was. They are obese, ridden with guilt, tired, angry, and depressed, unable to find their way out of the maze of bad diet/bad results. But there *is* a way out. Part II of this book contains a plan that will help you change your eating habits so that you, too, can live a life of energy and health.

You are not made up of loose, unrelated parts. Rather, you operate as a wholly integrated system. Addictions to sugar keep you feeling disconnected from your body, your spirit, and your feelings. When you change the way you eat, you will change your life.

Aspartame

Aspartame is an artificial sweetener that combines two amino acids (aspartic acid and phenylalanine) that naturally occur in the body. Artificial combinations of these amino acids are advertised as natural, but when you add them to your diet, your nerve cells are more susceptible to degeneration. Degeneration occurs when the nerve cells are overworked and results in the cells literally falling apart and thus unable to function at their normal capacity. They are literally tired out from all the excess activity.

Aspartic acid is known as an excitotoxin because it excites the nerves to fire up and go to work. This is good because it keeps us alert. The problem comes when we have too much excitement. The body, in its infinite wisdom, has created a system comprised of the glial cells to compensate for this excess firing. These cells act as sponges, cleaning up excess excitotoxins. If the excitotoxin level is too high, however, the glial cells are incapable of absorbing the excess. Further, when nerve cells are excited over long periods of time, they can become damaged. This injury releases free radicals which compromise the health of all other cells. (Free radicals will be discussed in Chapter Nine.)

Christiane Northrup, M.D., writes in *Nutrition Action Health Letter* (April 1999) that over 6,000 foods contain aspartame. Does this strike you as an unbelievably high number? It did us. But when you go to the grocery store and look at the food labels, you will see that aspartame comes in colas, yogurt, hot chocolate mixes, gum, breath savers, and most anything that says "sugar free." Educate yourself about aspartame. We are not only addicted to refined carbohydrates, we are addicted to excitotoxins. Aspartame influences your mood and behavior just as caffeine and low blood sugar do. It's important to remember that aspartame is an artificial chemical that not only sweetens our food, but also causes us to crave more.

Symptoms of too much aspartame can be:

- Headaches
- Complexion problems
- Weight gain
- Mood swings
- Hair loss
- Increased cholesterol
- Heart palpitations

- Memory loss

If you are experiencing any of these symptoms, slowly decrease aspartame from your diet and see for yourself if the symptoms go away. (Getting off aspartame is covered in Part II.)

Jill was a high school math teacher. Her job was stressful and so was her home life. After taking care of her family, she had papers to grade and lessons to plan. She started drinking diet cola at lunch and within a year; she was drinking six a day. She had constant, dull headaches that aspirin usually relieved. She came to see Kathleen about the weight she had gained. Since her diet hadn't changed, she could not figure out why this was happening. When Kathleen suggested that the diet cola might be the problem, Jill said she would be willing to do without it for a while to see if this was the case. Shortly after she stopped drinking the colas, she called Kathleen. "Jill was fearful because she felt shaky and her head was pounding," Kathleen recalls. "She told me that every joint in her body was painful and that she was very tired."

Jill soon came to realize that aspartame was indeed addictive and that she was experiencing withdrawal. With support, she made it and to her delight, her headaches went away, she could think clearly, and she started to lose the weight she had gained.

Caffeine

Coffeehouses are sprouting up everywhere and are great places to socialize without alcohol. We can easily stop in any time of the day or night and get our java fix. Coffee comes hot and comforting or cold and refreshing, and it's sold in a variety of flavors and sizes.

Caffeine was discovered in coffee in 1820, and in tea around 1827. Scientifically speaking, caffeine is an addictive drug, pure and simple. You can experience the same effects from caffeine that you would from other addictive drugs such as cocaine or nicotine. These include mood alteration, physical dependence, and physical withdrawal. The United States Food and Drug Administration does not include caffeine on its "generally recognized as safe" list, although it acknowledges no clear evidence of hazard at normal levels, according to Stephen D. Nugent, N.M.D., in *The Nugent Report* (January 1998).

The report also states that about 80% of all adults and 20% (and this number is growing) of children in the United States drink coffee, tea, or cola every day. The average daily intake of caffeine is about 400mg per person. Let's face it, the stuff makes us feel good and supports us in our stressful lifestyles. It keeps us alert. It improves hand, eye, and mind performance and verbal memory. These are all good, right? So what's the problem? Actually, the problems are many.

Caffeine also stimulates the brain and the adrenal glands to release epinephrine, the fight-or-flight hormone. This can cause increased blood pressure, increased respiratory rate (number of times you breathe in and out in a minute), and increased kidney function (the reason you urinate more when you drink beverages containing caffeine).

The numerous health risks of caffeine are:

- Urinary loss of magnesium, calcium, sodium, and potassium

- As little as 200mg of coffee per day (two cups of coffee) can increase risk for osteoporosis and cause leg cramps and jittery nerves

- High blood pressure

- Irritation of the bladder, frequency of urination, and burning sensation during urination

- Increased gastrointestinal symptoms (irritable bowel syndrome, ulcers, heartburn, reflux, and hiatal hernia)

- Sore breasts and increased fibrocystic breasts

- Serious nutritional deficiencies leading to osteoporosis and iron deficiency (a single cup of coffee can reduce iron absorption by 39%)

- Migraine headaches

And if this weren't enough, add adrenal stress, low blood sugar, mood and energy swings, insomnia, and depression. Women are more susceptible than men to these symptoms, because caffeine stays in their systems longer. And because it takes their bodies longer to metabolize caffeine, women are affected by smaller doses of caffeine than men.

How much caffeine are you taking in? Here are some numbers provided by Christiane Northrup, M.D., in *Health Wisdom for Women* (February 1999):

- Coffee = 100-150mg per 8 oz

- Tea steeped for three minutes = 28-50mg per 8 oz

- Hot cocoa = 30-50mg per 8 oz

- Cola drinks = 30-50mg per 12 oz can

- Milk chocolate = 6mg per oz

- Baking chocolate = 35mg per oz

- Anacin® (maximum strength) = 32mg per tablet

- Excedrin® = 64.8mg per tablet

Because caffeine is addictive and is found in so many foods that comprise our American diet today, it's not an easy matter to simply walk away from it. However, if you choose to clean your body of destructive toxins and eat only life-giving, nutrient-dense foods, caffeine will need to go. We'll show you how to detoxify from the effects of caffeine in Part II.

Decaffeinated Coffee

This brings us to the topic of decaffeinated coffee. People want to know if they can avoid all the problems listed above by just drinking decaffeinated beverages. The choice is up to you. Here are some facts to help you make your decision:

- Almost all decaffeinated coffee has some caffeine in it, usually around 3mg per cup.

- Pesticides are often found in the beans and do not get removed with processing.

- Coffee beans are treated with carcinogenic (cancer causing) substances to remove the caffeine. When you ingest these substances, the overtaxed liver has one more toxin with which to deal. The only safe method we know for removing caffeine from coffee is the chemical-free Swiss water method. The container must say, "decaffeinated by the Swiss water method" and not simply use catchy words like "naturally decaffeinated" or "water method used."

- The caffeine taken from coffee beans is usually sold to soft drink companies!

Is decaffeinated coffee harmful to you? Ask your body. Listen to its voice. Watch for signs to see if decaffeinated coffee agrees with you. Are you belching more after drinking it? Do you have more indigestion? Your body will speak to you.

Why Do I Still Desire These Foods?

As you start listening to your body and become more attuned to its messages, you are going to hear it saying that it wants fats, sugar, salt, and artificial sweeteners. If these foods are not always good for you, why then is your body craving them? There are many reasons.

As you learned in this chapter, these foods can start a chemical reaction in the body that results in an addiction that will set up additional chemical reactions that sustain the craving and cause it to steadily increase over time. Genetically, there is a primitive part of our brain that craves certain foods such as fat, sugar, and salt. We need a certain amount of fat, but the problem is that we have available to us an abundance of cheap, nutrient-deficient, saturated or trans-fatty acid food.

Also, sugar is sweet, and this is the taste our ancient ancestors used to determine if a new plant was safe to eat. They used their taste buds, intuition, and trial and error to determine if a plant was a food source, a medicine, or if it was unfit for human consumption or use. We are still programmed to like sweet tastes. The artificial sweeteners act like sugar in our system. Salt, on the other hand, enhances flavor.

From what we know of the history of salt, it was once a spice reserved for royalty. It was a status symbol, and in many ancient societies it was a form of currency. Salt's history, along with its ability to greatly enhance the flavor of food, makes it an inviting commodity. Salt is a normal chemical—electrolyte—in the body that must be balanced with other chemicals (especially potassium) in order for it to do its job. If we introduce too much salt into the diet, it is the responsibility of the kidneys to rid the body of the excess. In other words, too much salt unbalances the system and creates more work for the body and its organs, resulting in less energy and vitality and diminished health.

After World War II, a new and vast industry evolved whose sole purpose was to manufacture flavors. Even though this flavor business stays out of the public eye, it provides a very big part of our daily food intake. Most of the money that Americans spend on food is used to buy processed food. In the process of being "processed," these foods are depleted of their flavor and aroma. Research has shown that most of what we taste is determined by the gases that are released from food as we eat it. These gases flow up our nostrils and send signals to the brain that register flavor and taste to our tongue. Have you ever noticed when you have a cold and your nose is stopped up that you cannot taste your food? The people in the food and beverage industries have gotten very good at what they do. They know what flavors, smells, and textures will keep you coming back for more. They can take any food and turn it into a comfort food so that you will find pleasure every time you eat it. As far as they're concerned, food doesn't have to deliver nutrients, health, or vitality to your body. It only has to deliver pleasure. And when it does, you are hooked, for you are genetically programmed for pleasure. The fast-food business has relied heavily on the "flavor indus-try" to keep it profitable.

It's important to recognize our emotional connection to food. What we think our body wants may well be an emotional issue that we have not yet addressed. With practice, you will learn how to go beyond these emotional-based signals and discover what the deeper language of the body is telling you. Such "deeper language" may be experienced as gas and bloating, indigestion, headaches, constipation, diarrhea, depres-sion, moodiness, apathy, fatigue, and something as apparently simple as a general yucky feeling. What Kathleen's brother-in-law experienced is a good example.

He grew up in a typical Midwestern city and existed on a diet loaded with processed foods. Nothing unusual about that, he thought. Why, it was the modern thing to do! But he also experienced constant gas. That, too, he considered to be normal. When he finally changed his diet, however, and began replacing fast food and processed food with nutrient-dense and whole, natural foods, the gas diminished dramati-cally. Interestingly, when he returned home to visit his mother, he was fed his old childhood diet and the gas returned. He could then clearly see the direct correlation between what he ate and how he felt. He was finally able to understand what his body was saying to him. (In Part II, we will show you how you, too, can read and understand your body's language.)

What's Happening to Us?

We are eating super-sized meals and fast foods. Refined and processed foods have become a way of life for us. We take in large doses of sugar, chemicals and additives such as aspartame, caffeine, saturated fats, and trans-fatty acids. Our bodies are simply not programmed to deal with these substances. Instead of nutrients, our bodies have a toxic pool of chemicals and sugar with which to contend. The integrity of our immune system, our hearts, and other body functions are at risk for dis-ease. As you've learned from this chapter, we are what we eat. Food has a direct impact on the quality of our lives. Does it support your life, or does it diminish it? As you become more educated about foods and their effects on your body, you are better able to make positive choices.

Now that we have a better understanding of how food impacts our body, emotions and moods, let's look at another area that affects our connectedness or disconnectedness to our inner wisdom. Toxins have a direct impact on how we feel about ourselves. They can deplete the vitality we are trying to achieve.

9

Toxins and Your Body

Optimum health occurs in a clean and balanced body. Unfortunately, however, we encounter many kinds of toxins in our daily lives. Some are internal poisons and others come from the environment. It is useful to know something about these toxins and to understand how to rid your body of them.

Just as our heart beats nonstop and our lungs breathe automatically, our body's metabolic processes naturally dispose of toxins and poisons day in and day out. Some are cellular wastes that are toxic byproducts of metabolism, while others are pollutants and poisons that we take in through air, food, water, and the pores of our skin.

Under ideal circumstances, the body neutralizes and disposes of toxins through natural channels:

- Liver—neutralizes toxins or passes them out of the body through the digestive tract

- Kidneys—filter the blood, remove toxins through the urine, and regulate electrolytes

- Colon—removes solid food waste from the digestive system and excess toxins from the liver

- Lungs—this efficient filter eliminates carbon dioxide and other toxins from air pollution and gas from a toxic and congested bowel

- Skin—the largest organ of the body disposes of waste materials, particularly if the kidneys and colon are sluggish

- Lymphatic System—a network of vessels found in all body tissue through which lymph flows, removing dead cells, waste, large proteins, and bacteria from tissues

Our body's metabolic processes naturally dispose of toxins and poisons from our body. Just as you get ashes as waste from a fire, our bodies are constantly burning metabolically and creating waste for the body to dispose of. This waste from the metabolic process creates free radicals.

Free radicals are molecular thieves that have an "excited," unpaired electron in their outer shell, making them unstable. Free radicals steal electrons from other molecules in order to stabilize themselves. In the process, the "victim" molecule becomes a free radical, which in turn steals an electron from another molecule, which steals an electron from another molecule, and on and on.

As this electron transfer is vital to our life processes, our body has an antioxidant system that ensures that this transfer proceeds in a controlled manner. The antioxidant system is made up of vitamins, minerals, and enzymes that quench little metabolic fires at just the right time so that the free radicals will not get out of hand and cause cellular damage.

Unfortunately, in our industrialized world, this system can become overwhelmed by sources of oxidant stress including environmental pollution, petrochemical exposure and contamination, and unclean food sources.

Environmental Sources of Toxins

As we saw in Chapter Six, food production is one of the main sources of environmental toxins. Agricultural chemical residues and additives not only introduce toxins into the body, but they also lack the nutrients that the body needs in order to deal with toxins.

Water is the most important nutrient in the body and makes up two-thirds of the body's mass. Our drinking water is often recycled and can be filled with bacteria. In addition, despite stringent methods to prevent it, water is often contaminated with human excrement and chemicals. How thoroughly water is cleaned before it is recycled depends on the area in which you live and the quality control of your local water board. Most cities disinfect water with chlorine, and many also add sodium fluoride to help prevent tooth decay. But chlorine and fluoride can be harmful to our bodies.

Chlorine can be harmful in several ways:

- It combines with organic substances in water to form chloroform, a poisonous cancer-causing chemical.

- It destroys vitamin E.

- It destroys beneficial flora (bacteria) of the intestines.

- Sodium fluoride, too, can be damaging:

- It may inhibit functioning of the thyroid gland and enzyme systems.

- It may damage the immune system.

Fluoride occurs in some water naturally as calcium fluoride. However, hydrofluosilicic acid, a hazardous waste by-product of the phosphate fertilizer industries, is found in both water and toothpaste, according to Linda Page, N.D., in an article titled "Is Fluoride a Danger to Your Health and Sanity" which appeared in the *Holistic Times* (Vol. 5, Number 3, 1998). Small children are at greatest risk. The poison control centers located in large cities in the United States receive over 11,000 calls a year regarding people who have swallowed fluoride toothpaste and are experiencing vomiting and muscle cramps, both symptoms of fluoride poisoning.

Air Pollution

Every day, we breathe toxic fumes from traffic, cigarette smoke, tar, and other environmental sources—chemicals such as sulfur dioxide, carbon monoxide, nitrogen oxides, hydrocarbons, benzene, and lead. These and other pollutants are responsible for an increase in respiratory illnesses such as asthma, bronchitis, and chronic sore throats.

Environmental Illnesses

The medical profession acknowledges that there are environmental illnesses in which people working in sealed structures with re-circulated air can suffer a variety of ailments such as headaches, joint pain, nausea and vomiting, dizziness, and asthma-like symptoms. These illnesses are frequently referred to as "tight building syndrome" or "sick building syndrome" and can affect air travelers as well. New carpeting, chemical adhesives, toxic cleaning products, toxic fumes and gases emitted by petrochemical-based products, and volatile organic compounds in plywood and wallboard are also among the things that can trigger allergic responses and weaken the immune system.

Toxic Metals

We pick up toxic metallic elements from air, water, and food supplies, the most common of which are lead, arsenic, aluminum, and mercury. These toxins can remain in our bodies for an entire lifetime, wreaking havoc with our metabolic systems. Exposure to these can include such things as mercury from silver amalgam tooth fillings and aluminum from cookware, drinking water, baking powder, deodorant, antacid tablets, etc.

Radiation

Radiation can occur from nuclear fallout, X-rays, microwaves, high voltage power lines, television sets, computer monitors, clock radios, electric blankets, etc. Prolonged exposure to radiation contributes to aging, cellular distortion and abnormalities, leukemia and other forms of cancer, birth defects, anemia, and other diseases.

Drugs

Residues from medical and so-called "recreational" drugs often get stored in the liver, brain, and other tissues and create toxic by-products. A short list of these drugs includes alcohol, marijuana, tranquilizers, pain relief drugs, birth control pills, artificial hormone replacements, antibiotics, tobacco, and such steroid-type drugs as prednisone.

Parasites

The most common parasites in the United States are pinworms, round-worms, and tapeworms. One of the common ways to get these worms is from living with pets. Sleeping with pets and kissing them are two common ways that worms are transferred to humans. Other ways to get worms are by eating uncooked meat and fish, by not cleaning fruits and vegetables (even organic ones), walking barefoot in the dirt, and poor hygiene (such as not washing your hands before meals and after using the toilet). Some symptoms you might experience if you have parasites are weakness, significant weight loss, ravenous appetite, pale skin, itching of the rectum (especially at night), fretful sleep, and grinding teeth while sleeping.

Cosmetics, Shampoos, Hair Conditioners, Lotions, Shaving Creams

Many products that we use on a daily basis contain dyes, chemicals, and petrochemical-based substances that are absorbed through the skin.

The liver's job is to detoxify them. But if the liver is congested from toxic overload, these toxins can be transferred to other organs of elimination. Unfortunately, this process contributes to a polluted physical body.

Candles

This may come as a shock to you but, yes, even candles can be toxic. Many candles are made with paraffin, a petroleum by-product. When burned, it releases carcinogenic soot that can be taken in by the lungs. Also, most aromatherapy candles are scented with synthetic oils that release microscopic particles that can cause cancer and other health problems. Adding scents to candles often softens the wax, so the manufacturers sometimes use lead to make the wicks firmer. When burned, these wicks release lead into the air. Exposure to lead has been linked to hormone disruption, behavioral problems, learning disabilities, and numerous health problems. In Part II, we've listed places where you can purchase healthy candles.

Stress

This is a big one. Let's look at what stress creates on a physical level. Our lifestyles can often cause us to be hurried, frazzled, anxious, angry, and fearful. Biologically, stress puts our bodies in a "fight-or-flight" mode. When this happens, our adrenal glands release epinephrine which shuts down the digestive system and directs the blood to our muscles (to provide strength) and our brains (to provide quick thinking.) The "fight-or-flight" syndrome is essential if we need to run for our life or save our child from an oncoming car. But the "fight-or-flight" syndrome should not be necessary in order for us to function in our everyday world.

Stress weakens our system and adds to the effects of toxins and wastes already in the body. Constant repetition of a stressful situation puts strain on the adrenal glands and digestive system. Accumulated stress may also cause muscle tension, fatigue, anxiety, diarrhea, constipation, gas, reflux, and a listless feeling. Stress also weakens the power of the immune system to fight off illness. Toxins that build up in the body can quickly become too much for the immune system to properly handle.

The good news is that we can do something about it. In Part II, we will explain how to manage and reduce stress and how to avoid major environmental toxins.

The Holistic Definition of Disease

We have come to believe that disease is something that *happens to us*, that *we are victims* of it. We think that we have bad genes, that we caught a virus because someone coughed on us, or that we have a "bug" of some sort. But if we look at disease from a holistic mind, body, and soul perspective, then we can more clearly see that disease is really a breakdown and disharmony of the human organism.

Rich Work, in his book *Proclamations of the Soul,* does an excellent job of describing disease from a holistic point of view. He states that the cause of all chronic disease is disharmonious emotions, and he compares disease to a pyramid. The top of the pyramid is the disease. The next layers below it are tobacco, alcohol, toxic metals, pesticides and chemicals in our food and water, and all other sources of environmental toxins. The bottom layer of this pyramid, the base of it all, consists of toxic emotions.

We cover toxic emotions in more detail elsewhere in the book, but for now let us look at an example. Let's say that you are in an unhappy marriage or job, or perhaps you feel angry or bad about yourself. You stuff the feelings inside and keep saying, "I am sick and tired of this, but I will gut it out because _____." (Place your reasons in the blank.) Before long, you start to feel tired and maybe a little sick. If you continue to avoid your anger and tiredness, which are signals to pay attention to something, your immune system becomes compromised because of the internal stress. Toxins soon start to build up in your body which no longer has the energy to clear them away. Your body is assaulted by its own waste products.

You find yourself with increased colds, sinus infections, and other symptoms. You start going to the doctor more frequently. For a while at least, this pill and that antibiotic seem to help. With time, however, you find that they're helping less and less. Then you notice that your joints are starting to ache. You blame this on the aging process. All this gets in the way of that well-intentioned exercise program you started a while back. You try making yourself feel better or covering up your feelings by eating foods that lack nutrients and are toxic. Years go by, and now you have the big one—cancer or heart disease. Now you really are sick and tired, so much so that the illness gives you a way out from the job or marriage that you hated in the first place.

All of these are gradual processes, so gradual that we are often unaware that they are even occurring. Over a period of time, the malnourished and toxic body builds up to a chronic disease state. It tries to balance and stabilize itself, even in the midst of all the insults and onslaughts. True, the consequence of prolonged stress may just be feeling tired all the time. It may, however, escalate into a serious disease such as cancer.

Lisabeth's Journey

One of Kathleen's clients does an eloquent job of sharing her experience in learning this process of disease and the connectedness to self to find healing. Hers is a message of how disease is a step-by-step process—both into illness and out of it. She captures how one must deal with the body, emotions, and with the mind and spirit in order to truly heal, for it is when all are not working together in harmony that sickness most often begins. Here is Lisabeth's story in her own words.

"I don't have a long list of degrees, nor have I written any best-sellers. I've just been a passionate high school English teacher for twenty-three years, tucked away in my own little, private part of the world. My only claim to fame involves loving and being married to the same man for twenty-seven years and raising two responsible, adult children and...pause, deep breath...having walked the road of every woman's worst nightmare...Stage IV, metastasized, 'you better get ready to die,' breast cancer.

"The good news is that I have not only survived, but am thriving. My cancer markers are all in normal range and I'm all in one piece. True, I am no longer the saucy little brunette I used to be. Allowing myself to go gray represents the transformation of the trials, the testing, and the triumph, and serves as a daily reminder that I will no longer hide who I am or where I've been.

"In no way am I suggesting that anyone who may ever face such a challenge should disregard the potential severity and dangers of not seeking professional guidance. As a matter of fact, I sought professional guidance, too. It's just that it took a lot of time and a lot of doctors before I learned that I couldn't necessarily trust strangers to know what was best for my body. I had to take responsibility for myself. Through much trial and error, I eventually gathered a strong support system of a variety of health care practitioners which included holistic and naturopathic physicians, massage and reflexology therapists, colon hydrotherapists, nutritionists, a biological dentist, practitioners in energy medicine, biofeedback, acupuncture, and Chinese herbs, and most importantly, a supportive husband.

"What I am saying, above all else, is to trust your gut! The innate intelligence of your body is constantly sending you messages and working on your behalf. That still, quiet voice from within won't lead you astray; but you'll have to turn down the volume on the static that keeps intruding. The static is often in the form of someone else's fear, and I had enough of my own fear. Taking on anyone else's fear of cancer only compounded my own.

"I still remember the look on the face of the woman who did my mammogram for the fourth time that day, just to make sure she had it 'right.' Her face said it all. I remember the doctor who, after doing the ultrasound, told me, it was indeed a mass.

"I remember the certified letter from that woman surgeon who told me that I would die if I didn't submit to immediate surgery. I remember the surgeon of whom I asked, 'Where did this come from? What caused it? How much time do I have to decide?' I knew I was in the wrong place when she shrugged all my questions away with her honest and forthright reply, 'I don't know. I'm just trained to cut.'

"I remember trying to bravely teach before five classrooms full of teenagers each day, when in fact I was living in total fear—fear of dying, fear of pain and suffering, fear of perhaps having to have my femininity sliced from my body. I remember the look on the X-ray technician's face as she tried to calmly tell me that they are making arrangements to admit me to the hospital at once. Fluid had filled my chest cavity because of tumors everywhere, the size of fifty-cent pieces.

"I remember the young intern who took my medical history while checking her nail polish, chomping on her gum, and unconsciously kicking her crossed leg. I remember the team of young residents who could only offer chemotherapy for palliative pain relief but no cure. They did, however, provide the phone number of a hospice agency and they did offer assistance in creating a living will. I looked at my husband and told him with my eyes, 'Let's get out of here.'

"My holistic doctor said it was time to go to Mexico. Initially, I was going to have insulin potentiation therapy. A doctor in Tijuana could administer it…creating a hypoglycemic state in the body and when the body is starved for glucose, tag it with small doses of chemotherapy. I remember sitting on the examination table, breaking into tears, saying to my husband, 'I can't do that. This isn't right for me.'

"An acquaintance of a very good friend—with a tumor the size of a football on her kidney had also gone to Mexico and was treated by another doctor in Tijuana. She's been in remission now for six years. I remember conjuring up all these negative images of what Tijuana must be like. I was wrong, very wrong. At my friend's suggestion, I phoned her doctor in Mexico.

"He returned the call and must have spent an hour talking with my husband and me. He talked of breast cancer…failure of the endocrine system…my body being different from everyone else's…no two cancers alike. He is an oncologist and an immunologist, trained in the United

States, a Ph.D. in metabolic therapy, and with impeccable worldwide credentials. My kind of guy!

"My husband and I headed south of the border to find and entrust my life to this man. I remember when he took my husband aside after confirming that the disease was in my liver. 'Do we tell her?' Of course. 'Are you ready for the fight of your life? I'll do my part, and we'll leave the rest to God.' Immune therapy…sixteen days of IV's. Detoxify the body first and above all else, do no harm to the body, and then begin killing the cancer cells while creating new healthy cell memory. Rest. Vaccine therapy, live cell biological therapy, herbal and metabolic support, as well as oxygen therapy. Coffee enemas. Fresh juices. Walks to the ocean. The sounds of Sara Brightman and Andrea Bocelli recordings wafting through our room. Daily calls from our daughter in New York City and prayers from family, friends, and from people I didn't even know. Tears. Night sweats…dreams, full of rage…a lifetime of stored, repressed anger in my liver, detoxing. Three-hour visits by the doctor each day and a personal protocol just for me, my body type, and my type of cancer. There were therapies from all over the world that represented truly integrative medicine—the best of both worlds of conventional medicine and natural therapies. And a doctor who knew exactly what he was doing.

"Home in time for Christmas. A personal protocol just for me…continue the vaccines and the metabolic and herbal programs that had been started in the hospital. I was taking hourly pills starting at 7:00 A.M. until 10:00 P.M. each day. I had monthly blood tests. Before we left for Tijuana, my last X-ray showed that my own immune system had created a 'bolus' in my left lung, completely encasing all the tumors into a ball. My body, having now been given the chance, was ready to rid my body of this disease.

"My husband and I then attended a week-long program, an intensive exploration into all the negative, generational patterning we adopt as a means of getting love. I have to admit, my husband was more willing than I to face the complex, emotional component that led us both into the crisis of our lives.

"By February, my lungs and liver were completely clear, although I still have a residual tumor in my breast that has calcified. I am continuing with my intensive regime and am on my way to renewed and revitalized health, knowing full well that true healing takes time. It's essential that I realize, however, that it's not about fixing, perfecting, or disciplining myself in an effort to defeat death. It's about relaxing, and relishing in the fact, that just as Hamlet says, 'The readiness is all.' Those who say it can't be done shouldn't interrupt those doing it.

"I believe in a God who is intimately aware of each one of us, and has a uniquely designed plan for us all. Cancer has been my gift—one that has transformed me forever, bringing me into the realization that everything that happens, good and bad, is for our benefit, ultimately bringing a channel of blessing."

As Lisabeth's story shows, the good news is that we *can* be in charge of our health and well-being. By altering our thoughts and behavior, we can change our physical organism. As Caroline Myss, Ph.D., the author of books on this subject has said, "Your biography is your biology." You can learn to support your body by keeping it clean and nourished. You can control the outcome of your health more than you thought possible. In Part II, you will learn how to listen to your body and how to clean it up.

II

Introduction

When we welcome all of our emotional experiences, we begin to enter the unified world of the body, mind, and spirit. It is our emotions that are in reality our guidance system directing us on the path to wholeness and health.

Dr. Candace Pert, in her book *Your Body Is Your Subconscious Mind*, found that our body's opiate receptors—those molecular-level receiving stations that take in information and respond by issuing to us messages of bliss—while densely concentrated in the brain, also occur in every other part of the body. The implication is that emotions are not generated by the brain, but by the cells themselves! Since these receptor-bearing cells reside all over the body, blissful experiences and all other emotions occur in the blood, organs, muscles, tissues, and bones at the same time as they are registered in the brain. The "limbic" part of the brain then transfers the information to the brain's frontal cortex, and it is only at this point that we become conscious of the emotion and begin to form ideas about what we're feeling. The experience itself actually occurs at a pre-conscious, physiological level. This is even further proof that our emotions are truly our body's messages to us. They are our direct connection to our inner wisdom and body intelligence.

If you are committed to being in touch with your body wisdom, you must learn to embrace your emotions. Being in touch with your emotions begins by being able to identify your feelings accurately as soon as possible after you've had them. As you progress, you will be able to name and recognize your feelings in real time. To say that you're angry is a simple example of being able to identify in the moment how you are feeling. When you recognize your true feelings, you can then deal with them effectively. Sometimes that will mean actually speaking them out, sometimes it will not. If you don't recognize and process your feelings, however, you are likely to act them out in some other way. (Slamming a door or ignoring someone who is talking to you are examples of acting out emotions.) Some long-term results of being disconnected from your feelings are: dysfunctional relationships at home or work, over- and under-eating, addictions, emotional and/or physical abuse (giving or receiving), and physical illness.

Unexpressed feelings often appear as illness. It may seem as though you suddenly came down with a cold; but long before your first symptoms appeared, your body sent you numerous messages that some corrections were needed. When those signals were neither heard nor heeded, your body began to break down, and eventually you became ill. Other common messages from your body are headaches, body aches, moodiness, and lethargy. These are just a few of the feelings that serve as bridges between your health and your spiritual wellness. Learning to recognize and to tend to these early symptoms is a major step towards actively loving yourself.

Our feelings are the barometers of what is going on inside us physically, mentally, emotionally, and spiritually. If we cut ourselves off from our feelings, it's like tearing the rudder off a boat—we can still float, but we have no way of steering.

We have designed Part II of this book to guide you through exercises that will help you get connected to your feelings. We've included stories of how others have used their feelings as bridges to wholeness and health, and also information that will help you experience positive feelings regarding your body and your relationship with food. Part II covers:

- How to finally break the relentless cycle of unexpressed feelings and repeated patterns

- How to identify unique ways of finding satisfaction and maintaining peace and balance in your life

- How to navigate a successful relationship between your feelings and your food
- How to "detox" from foods and activities that dull your sensitivity to your feelings

10

Real Satisfaction

When it comes to food, the only real satisfaction comes from being in the present moment with your mind, your body, whatever you are eating, and allowing yourself to feel satisfied with the experience. That satisfaction is essential to having a *Full Heart/Satisfied Belly*! True satisfaction means not having to wait until something else happens in order for you to be happy. Real satisfaction means not having to say, "Well, that was pretty good, but what I really wanted was _____," (you fill in the blank).

Satisfaction appears when you come down from the "moon palace of myths and longing" and enter the real world and begin listening to what your body is telling you. In order to hear and heed those messages, it is imperative that you become aware of the current moment that you learn to truly live in and savor the present.

There are many ways to practice the art of being in the present moment. Meditation, being aware of your breathing, focusing acutely on your surroundings, and mindful eating are just a few of your options. When you are emotionally satisfied in the present moment and not using food as a substitute for fulfillment, your consciousness and energy will be available for other aspects of your life.

Mindful eating is a great place to start practicing being in the present, because you get to practice at least three times a day! There are other benefits, too. When you begin to make a habit of feeling satisfied with the food you eat, you will begin to relax inside. Eventually, your body will adjust to its natural weight (*i.e.*, the amount, within a few pounds up or down that you weigh without dieting or trying to gain weight).

There is, however a cost to achieving real satisfaction. You have to give up the habit (by some mistakenly considered a luxury) of unconsciously eating whatever you want, whenever you want. That sense of being able to eat without the limitations of conscience is what people often do when they are on vacation. For some, it's a ritual!

Are you dissatisfied with some aspect of your life, or perhaps your life in general? If so, do you feel powerless to do something about it? Do you occasionally express your frustration by overeating? Be honest now, do you have a rebellious voice inside of you that sometimes says, "No one is going to tell me what and when to eat! I eat *what* I darn well please, *when* I darn well please!" Choosing to be truly satisfied in each and every present moment means that you have to learn to listen to that feisty inner voice and ask it what it really wants. You will quickly discover that food is totally ineffective at helping you become connected to yourself, someone else, the earth, or your own spirit. When you are craving such connections, food will never fill you up!

When your primary way of feeling connected has been through food, making a conscious decision to eat differently is likely to feel a little scary, as though you're giving up something that has been a valuable part of your life. This is how one of Linda's clients worked though the process of becoming aware of his eating habits and discovered the benefits of mindful eating.

Robert was an architect who ate junk food because it was quick and easy. He kept potato chips, crackers, and pretzels in his desk drawer and munched on them through out the workday. A real meal for Robert was Chinese food—usually cashew chicken with white rice—delivered to his studio. Most of the time, he ate it right out of the box. Robert ate to give his body fuel, and was only barely tuned in to how the food tasted. Day after day, he ordered the same food out of simplicity and habit. Although he didn't take the time to exercise, he wasn't overweight. In fact, he had no real health challenges.

Then Robert met Diane, and they fell deeply in love. Diane loved to cook healthy foods and quickly introduced Robert to tastes he'd never encountered. They began hiking and rock climbing together. To his dismay, Robert discovered Diane had twice the energy he did. In her backpack, she brought organic fruit, nuts and seeds, and lots of water. Robert, on the other hand, packed his potato chips, candy bars, and bottles of cola. Through a misguided sense of machismo, he hid the fact that he was exhausted by the end of their treks. He silently vowed to begin exercising immediately.

Whenever Diane suggested he try some of her organic food, Robert became defensive about his lifelong eating habits. Here is a snapshot of some of Robert's thoughts and reactions, in chronological order over the period of a year, as he made the gradual change to mindfully eating higher quality foods:

- Diane is a health food nut. I will never eat that stuff!

- When she orders fish or tofu, I order french fries and a burger.

- When I'm at her house, I guess I have to eat what she serves, but when she's at my house, I'm putting steaks on the grill!

- No way am I going to give up my potato chips and Chinese food.

- Where does she buy all this health food anyway?

- All this organic food costs way too much money, as far as I'm concerned.

- She brought the lunch on our last trip and you know what? It was actually delicious!

- She challenged me to eat better food for a month and see how I feel. Okay, I did it. I have to admit that by week four, I felt better than I have for a long time. But as far as I'm concerned, it's still too much trouble to do everyday.

- Even though I am exercising now on a regular basis, I still can't keep up with Diane.

- It's hard to eat good food. There aren't any fast-food restaurants for that kind of food and what's worse, no one delivers!

- Okay, I can do it on the weekends. But it's too much trouble to do it everyday, especially when I'm working.

- I just noticed that there is a refrigerator in my office. I guess I could bring my lunch to work.

- I have to admit that when I eat healthy food for lunch, I don't get tired in the afternoons like I used to.

- Diane and I had an incredible meal at her house last night. She taught me about this thing called "mindful eating." I can't believe I never really enjoyed eating before. What a pleasure I have been missing!

- When I really slow down and eat mindfully, I'm surprised how greasy my Chinese food is. Honestly, now when I eat it slowly, it really doesn't taste very good. But I'm not ready to tell Diane that. She'll say, "I told you so," and I don't want to hear it!

- I went to a fast-food restaurant and got a hamburger. When I tasted it, I didn't like it. In fact, it was disgusting! You won't believe this, I threw it away!

- Diane and I found an oriental restaurant that uses less oil and MSG, and steams their vegetables. I'm now trying to eat all my food mindfully. If it tastes good and feels fulfilling in my body, I know I have a hit.

- I can't believe it myself! I now have soybean nuts in my drawer instead of potato chips. I have almonds instead of pretzels. I love those crunchy snacks! I have organic juice and fruit in the refrigerator and delicious chicken salad I picked up at the health food store. I have to put my name on everything; otherwise my coworkers will eat it before I do!

- Today I had an apple for a snack between breakfast and lunch. Later, when I went outside to the picnic table and ate my lunch, I watched the birds and squirrels play in the trees while I mindfully enjoyed every morsel of my food. I feel better than I have my whole life and can you believe it? I'm getting more work done than ever, too, even when I take forty-five minutes for lunch.

- Diane and I went on a hike yesterday and for the first time, I not only kept up without any problems, I was able to go ahead of her! Life is good!

Robert gradually changed the way he related to food. If he had tried to do everything at once, he would most likely have rebelled and there would have been no real change. As it was, he was able to move through his feelings and his behavior at his own tempo and come to new decisions based on how he felt, rather than on what he thought Diane wanted him to do. The practice of "mindful eating" was a major experience for Robert, because he was so used to always doing something else, like working on his computer or watching television, while he ate. Before, he seldom actually appreciated or enjoyed the food he was eating. Here is the ten-step mindful eating experience that Diane taught Robert:

1. Take the food you are going to eat and place it in front of you and look at it. Take your time and notice the colors. Pick it up and smell it. Think about where it came from—a field, a tree, or an animal. Bless the food, the energy of life that created it, and all the people who helped bring this food to you.

2. Thoughtfully decide what you want to taste first. With your utensil, take your first bite, and then put down your fork or spoon, and fully concentrate on that mouthful of food. Chew it slowly. Decide if you like it. If you don't like it (or it is just

okay), don't take a second bite. If you do like it, savor it. Be fully aware of the food in your mouth. If you find your thoughts going to the next bite or the next kind of food you plan to eat, bring your thoughts back to the present moment and the food that is in your mouth. No matter how hungry you are, chew your food slowly and allow yourself to enjoy it fully.

3. When you have swallowed that first bite, consciously decide what you will try next. Now pick up your utensil and slowly taste and enjoy that next bite. Once again, put your utensil down while you are chewing.

4. Notice how the food feels in your body as you swallow it. Relax your shoulders and your neck. Breath deeply, be present to your entire experience of eating.

5. Be aware of how the food tastes and the texture it has. Notice if it is crunchy or smooth. Be aware of how it feels and what tastes best to you right now. Be aware of your teeth, your tongue, and your lips. Are your taste buds excited?

6. Continue to eat in this mindful way, putting your utensil down between each bite, and making sure you're not eating anything you don't like.

7. If you are eating vegetables like carrots, eat just one at a time. If you decide you want more of something, feel free to get some more, but be sure to eat it in the same mindful way.

8. Throughout this exercise, notice how full (or satisfied) your stomach is feeling.

9. Quit eating when you begin to feel full, instead of eating until you are stuffed.

10. Take the time to become aware of how you feel physically, emotionally, and mentally.

Mindful eating can become a habit that you practice on a regular basis. As you begin this focus, however, you may find that you are not able to do all ten items every time. If that's the case, here are a few tips that are especially helpful when you're working. If you are eating at your desk, turn off the computer and put your phone on hold so you won't have to answer it while you're eating. If possible, turn your back to your workspace and focus on something other than your desk. Allocate a certain amount of time for yourself (even fifteen minutes will help). Focus on what you are eating and chew slowly. Let this time be a real break in which you are conscious of what you are eating and how you are feeling. Even if it is only a short bit of time, you will become conscious of what you have eaten and you will feel refreshed.

Even when you're at home or on the road, you may feel rushed. Therefore, we challenge you to:

- *Stop eating over the sink.* Sit down and focus on your food, even if you are in a hurry. Honor yourself by taking a few moments to simply be aware of chewing your food. When we eat in a hurry, we have a tendency to overeat. Your body needs twenty minutes before it registers you are full. When you are eating quickly, you can consume great quantities of food in a short amount of time. As a result, you feel stuffed and uncomfortable. Slow down! There's no hurry. You and your body will feel better with smaller portions of food.

- *Stop eating in front of the television.* This is one of the most common, mindless activities Americans do every day. The television has practically become a kitchen appliance! For many, the couch in front of the television has replaced the kitchen table. When you eat while doing something else, you cannot be fully attuned to how your food tastes or how full your body is feeling. Your enjoyment is reduced because you are doing two things at once. Also, this habit of eating in front of the television inhibits conversation. A meal is a special, sacred time when family and friends can share with each other stories of their daily activities.

Even though it may seem like it sometimes, your television set is *not* part of your family!

- *Stop eating while you are driving.* Talk about multitasking! Munching away while you're behind the wheel is the ultimate of a dangerous dual focus. It is just another mindless way to stuff yourself without nourishing yourself. Besides everything else that's been mentioned in this section, eating while driving puts your life (and the lives of others) in danger. For a much healthier and safer practice, try taking twenty more minutes before you leave for work to feed yourself. What if it does mean you have to get up twenty minutes earlier? If you're really interested in making peace with your body, that twenty minutes will pay off double-time!

Mindful eating has many components. It begins by noticing where you are when you're unconsciously eating, and by noticing the times you're eating when you're not even hungry or don't like the food. As you become more aware of those types of experiences, you can begin to make different choices. Mindful eating is one of the most valuable and really satisfying choices you will ever make. To eat mindfully on a regular basis, you may find it necessary to break some old habits. In the next chapter, we'll show you how to uproot those old beliefs and break that cycle of bad habits once and for all.

11

Breaking the Cycle

Linda recently put together a support group for making peace with your body. She asked the participants to share stories about their most successful experiences with breaking the cycle of negative beliefs and behavior. Everyone in the room just stared at her. She could tell by the looks on their faces that they were struggling to examine past behaviors from the viewpoint of success. Their first learning for that evening had already begun. They soon realized that they had been focusing on what hadn't worked, instead of on what had been successful. Here are a few of the success stories they shared.

Marcia

"I decided I wanted to look good for my high school reunion that was six months away. I followed a healthy food plan and began working out with a trainer three times a week. By the time I went to the reunion, I looked and felt better than I had since I was in high school. I was really proud of myself! I must have heard from a dozen of my classmates how good I looked. I was high for a month afterwards."

Sarah

"I began having a terrible rash and nothing seemed to stop the persistent itching. An allergist finally discovered I was allergic to chocolate. I was devastated to learn I was a 'chocoholic!' However, I stopped eating it to end the itching. It worked. And every time I even think about eating chocolate, all I have to do is remember how badly I itched and the craving instantly disappears!"

Frank

"I never ate breakfast, because I very seldom felt hungry when I woke up. Plus, since I had a tendency to sleep too long in the morning, I always felt like I was short on time. I figured I would take sleep over food any day! In any case, I was starved by noon and would wolf down a huge lunch. Eventually, I gained weight and began to feel disgusted with the way I looked. I tried several diets, with limited success. But no matter what I did, I never ate breakfast. Finally, after reading an article in a men's magazine about why breakfast is important in order to begin metabolizing the food for the day, I forced myself to get out of bed and eat something. I have been amazed at how much better I feel eating a healthy breakfast every day! Lunch is now normal-sized and, without having to make any other changes, I have actually lost a few pounds."

Rochelle

"I managed to not eat sugar for eighteen months."

Bob

"I'm intimidated by how successful you all have been. The best I've ever been able to do is to take a walk instead of eating a bag of potato chips!"

Doris

"On several occasions, I've been able to follow a strict diet for a couple of months. Each time, I lost fifteen pounds."

All of these people were proud of their accomplishments and fully deserved to be. But there was another reason Linda wanted them to focus on their ability to overcome challenges, and that's because success leaves clues. When we are so busy looking at our mistakes or how we dropped the ball, we miss the value of our own personal markers of success. Sometimes, we need help from someone else to point out what we have done right. And even if it is only once that we broke out of our pattern of negative thoughts and behavior, it still counts! It may not be enough, but it's a beginning.

Take credit for that victory. We all need encouragement along the way!

Along with the successes these people had, however, there was another side to their stories.

Marcia

"Well, yes, I did lose all that weight for the reunion; but when I came home and was so high from all the compliments I had gotten, I started my old habit of celebrating with food. At first, I told myself I deserved it. After a while, however, I couldn't stop myself. After six months of hard work. I was absolutely sure I would never gain an extra pound, I gained all the weight back—and more! I was more ashamed of myself than ever, and I've been beating myself up ever since. This support group is the first thing I've tried since I gained the weight back a year ago."

Sarah

"It's true that I have avoided chocolate because of that rash. What I didn't tell you was that I have found a substitute that doesn't cause me to itch but still satisfies my sweet tooth. The bad part is that I'm now eating ice cream by the gallons. I can't believe I haven't gained any weight! My cholesterol, however, is sky high. The doctor says I'm a candidate for a heart attack, and I'm only thirty-seven years old! She also says I need to cut back on fats and sugar, but I haven't been able to last any more than a day without my fix of ice cream."

Frank

"So far, I have continued to eat breakfast for sixty days in a row. I'm proud of that, but I'm also a little nervous about how I will handle the time that will inevitably occur when I don't eat breakfast. Will that start up my old poor eating habits again? I've always been a bit of an extremist about everything my whole life.

If I fall off the wagon, so to speak, can I get back on without trashing my success?"

Rochelle

"It was really weird! After eighteen months of successfully avoiding sugar, I went to my cousin's birthday party and as they cut the cake, I had this overwhelming desire to have a piece like everybody else. I did hear my inner wisdom say that I wasn't even hungry, but that old rebel part of me was particularly powerful that day. It was as if I heard it whisper in my ear, 'Why do I have to be the only one not eating cake and ice cream? It doesn't seem to hurt anyone else! I want it and I'm going to have it!' I ate that piece of cake so fast I barely tasted it. What I do remember was finding the heavy sweetness repulsive. But I ate it anyway! It was several days later in my therapy session with Linda before I finally figured out what was really going on with me."

Bob

"My problem is boredom. The reason I mentioned that I was successful in taking a walk instead of eating a bag of potato chips was because it was the only time so far that I've been able to distract myself from eating out of boredom by doing something else. I wish I had more positive experiences to report. So far, that's my only one."

Doris

"What I have learned about myself is that when I feel totally out of control in my life, I have to get a grip on something or I think I'll go crazy. Oddly enough, those are the times I've been the most successful with dieting. I now know that it's because I channeled all my desire to control something into being very strict with my food. It feels good, because I have the illusion of having control over at least one aspect of my life (for a month or so, anyway!). I'm finally learning that I allow my life to spin out of control because I am so afraid of conflict. I know that's my real issue. When I feel that I'm being taken advantage of, I overeat. Then I feel even worse! At that point, I'm taking advantage of myself! When that happens, I put myself on a strict diet in order to regain control. It's been an endless cycle my entire life, but it's one I'm dedicated to breaking!"

That same night, the members of this support group talked more about the major connections between emotions and food. Marcia, for example, revealed that she was more concerned about how she looked to others than she was about being genuinely motivated to change her negative thoughts and beliefs about herself. She could finally see that she was doing exactly as the advertisers and media wanted her to do. She was buying into the "quick fix" approach. And when the "quick fixes" failed, as they almost always do, she assumed that it was she who had failed. If she had not chosen to come to a support group, she most likely would have continued on her well-worn path of diet and disappointment and back to diet again. There is the prevalent idea—again, perpetuated by the advertisers and the media—that we can quickly and painlessly and without any effort whatsoever change how our bodies look and do so without attending to our underlying feelings and habits. Making real and lasting changes, however, requires consistent motivation and long-term commitment.

Marcia would eventually have to examine those issues for herself and perhaps have to face the truth that she may not be sufficiently motivated to consistently look like she did at the reunion. She can still find a level of motivation, however, that works for her and brings her to a higher level of health. Marcia will be healthier by staying at a heavier consistent weight than by continuing the repetitious pattern of weight loss and weight gain.

Sarah's life and relationships were subtly beginning to spin out of control. Her allergy was brought on because she had used chocolate as a substitute for the companionship of friends and the attention of a lover, both of which she craved. When chocolate was no longer a viable option, she just transferred her addiction to ice cream. Neither chocolate nor ice cream, however, was capable of solving her problem of loneliness. In the support group, Sarah was by far the most introverted participant. Although she had a hard time talking about herself, she was an excellent listener. Since she'd had so few friends in her life up to that point, she'd never before heard people share how they really felt. Little by little, Sarah began to open up and tell the others in the group about her self-imposed isolation and her fear of not being able to communicate with other people. As the evening progressed, she began to feel safe within the group and eventually showed everyone her wonderful self of humor! Bolstered by her experience in the support group, she began to open up at work as well. Eighteen months after beginning the support group, Sarah was still introverted, but she did have two new, close friends with whom she did fun activities. She also planned a small gathering at her apartment and had gone out on two dates. Ice cream was no longer her best friend and her cholesterol was down twenty points.

It was scary for Sarah to even agree to start coming to the group, but it was the best decision she could have made. When she began, she was unable to identify the fact that loneliness was her central issue. But as soon as she discovered what was really motivating her from inside, she was able to have a number of options besides ice cream.

When Frank described himself as an "all-or-nothing" kind of guy, that was a tip-off to his real control issues. When he followed a routine, you could count on him sticking to it, because it reassured him and made him feel as though he were in control. That's why he had been so successful with eating breakfast regularly. If he wavered just the tiniest bit from his breakfast schedule, his control was all gone! Frank was forced to examine just how rigid his way of controlling himself had become. His father was a military man and had schooled him in the benefits of following a predetermined routine. Frank, however, had carried that lesson to an extreme. His father also felt that if you weren't working, you were lazy. During his childhood, there had been no time for Frank to simply enjoy being a kid and relax. Even as a grown man, Frank had to fight himself to let go and have a good time. His moments of "rebellion" were those in which he slept until the last minute before he had to go to work, something that he'd never been allowed to do as a child.

When he gave up sleeping in and started eating breakfast, he felt much better. Naturally, there came a time when he did sleep too long and he missed his usual breakfast. His challenge at that point was not to overreact and completely give up on what he had discovered to be a healthy habit. Because he had been in the support group for a while, we had been able to prepare him for that possibility. On the morning he overslept, he had a piece of fruit while he was waiting for the elevator and a breakfast bar as soon as he got to his office. It wasn't his ideal meal, but it was far better than falling into his old rut of not eating at all. Frank was eventually able to check in with his inner wisdom to see if he needed to sleep in a little longer from time to time; but even on those occasions, he made it a point not to skip eating breakfast no matter what!

Most of the time, the way we eat has very little to do with food or hunger. Eating or not eating are commonly symptoms of another issue.

In Rochelle's case, she was puzzled by the fact that she'd eaten the birthday cake when she wasn't hungry and didn't even like that kind of cake. As we began to examine how she was feeling that day, however, it began to make sense. Having just gone through a divorce, Rochelle was understandably feeling disconnected. To make matters worse, she'd also been mourning the fact that she'd not yet had a baby. It just so happened that there were a lot of pregnant women and young children at the birthday party she attended. Rochelle was instantly miserable! She wanted to leave immediately. Instead, she did what she rationalized was socially correct—she stayed and tried to ignore her feelings or otherwise she felt she would burst into tears right in the middle of the birthday party! Stuffing down those feelings became momentarily easier when she was offered a big piece of sweet cake. With the help of the support group, Rochelle realized how her feelings that day had precipitated the whole series of events culminating in eating cake she didn't even like. Once she acknowledged those feelings, we could focus on the real issues of her sense of loss and mourning that were quite appropriate and needed to be dealt with emotionally, instead of with food.

Bob has just recently begun to examine the relationship between his emotions and his eating habits. Until the group experience, he had never even linked the two together. Boredom was Bob's constant and familiar companion. It was so normal, in fact, that it was hard for him to even identify at first. His parents had also been sedentary, quiet people who were generally blasé about life, so boredom seemed pretty natural to Bob. In order for Bob to change his couch potato habits, he had to find something fun to do that motivated him. He hated exercise. He was socially immature. His wife had stopped having any meaningful conversations with him because he was unable or unwilling to relate to her feelings or life experiences. When Bob heard what the others in the group had to say about their lives, he was astounded. He began to realize he was missing a great deal by substituting television, beer, and potato chips for social companionship and by forcing his wife away from him.

Bob slowly started to examine the fears he harbored about never being good enough and about communicating with others. Hesitantly at first, Bob learned to talk to the other members of the group. He role-played conversations with them and learned to accept their feedback, even when it wasn't positive. He made a list of activities he thought he might like to experience, and decided to begin by learning how to play bridge. His wife was astounded by his behavior! One evening, he surprised and delighted her by inviting her to go for a walk with him. From then on, their lives began to shift into positive possibilities. For starters, they decided to leave the television off during dinner and begin focusing on one another.

When Bob first came to the group, he thought it was to improve his physical health. And while that did happen, his ability and willingness to communicate on a personal level were an added bonus.

Doris had already discovered some of her major control issues before she joined the group. However, knowing why you do something and then not doing it anymore are two distinctly different things. It took Doris awhile to realize that fear was at the root of a lot of her problems. She had grown up with family members who constantly yelled at one another and had frequent and fearful arguments. As a little girl, she had been terrified.

By the time she was an adult, Doris was conditioned to believe that anytime she stood up for herself or disagreed with someone, a conflict (similar to the ones she'd witnessed as a child) would invariably ensue. As a result, she would go to great lengths to avoid any form of dissent. Eventually, her whole life started spinning out of control as her defense mechanisms tried to protect her more and more. The support group was a place for Doris to see how others were able to successfully manage conflict in ways much different than those used in her family. In the group, she saw people occasionally get upset with each other without yelling. Over time, she was able to let others in the group know when she, too, was upset. Everyone knew Doris was well along in her recovery when she expressed her irritation to Linda for allowing the group to continue ten minutes longer than usual! As Doris progressed, she was able to balance her eating with her nutritional needs without either eating everything in sight or putting herself on a very strict diet that she couldn't possibly maintain.

From the experiences of this group of people, you can see that breaking the cycle of eating-related habits is seldom just about the food. Key issues of control, rebellion, boredom, and other areas of conflict in your life must be examined. There is a process we all go through as we become aware of the challenges with which we are personally dealing. It's called the "Levels of Transformation." The next chapter will give you a road map of what you can expect as you progress along your own personal path of growth.

12

Levels of Transformation

Change of any kind can pose quite a personal challenge. In Linda's seminars and workshops, she often asks the people in her audiences how many of them have tried to change someone. Most of them raise their hands. Then Linda will ask of those with their hands up, how many of had succeeded in changing someone? At that point 99% of the hands go down. Of the few people who still have their hands up, she inquires, "Whom did you change?" Invariably, someone will answer, "Myself."

Yes, we can change ourselves. In fact, we are the only one we can change. To do so, however, requires commitment, motivation, and dedication. In doing so, there is a process we go through that allows us to see where we are on the path of personal development. We call this model:

Levels of Transformation

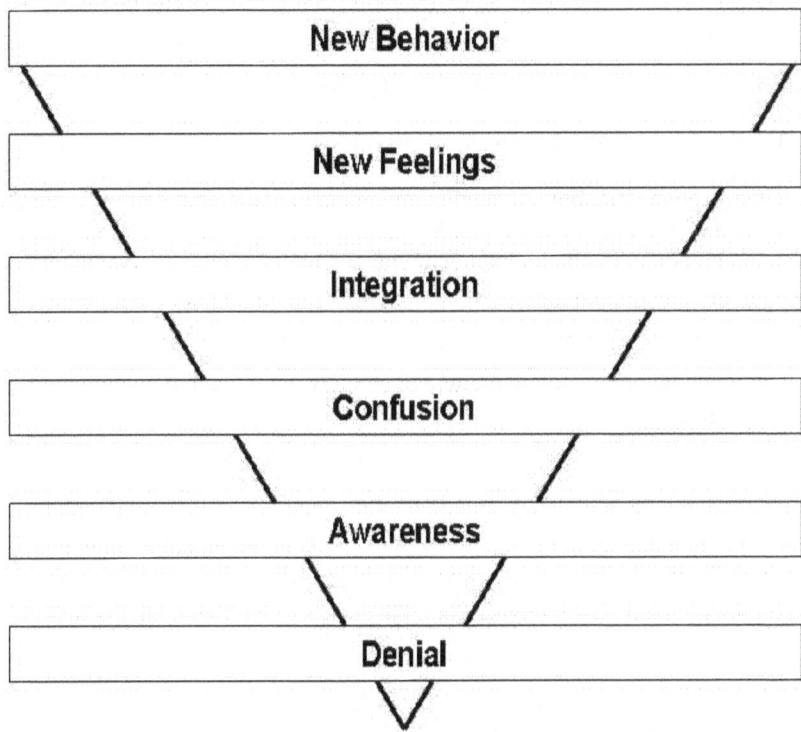

Denial is the first of the Levels of Transformation. Unfortunately, the vast majority of people in the United States seem to live and die in a constant state of denial. They are totally unaware of who they are, who they could be, and the possibilities that are available to them. As a result, they live in fear and apathy, never allowing themselves to know that they have the choice to think and feel differently. In order to stay in denial, a person must diligently practice these behaviors:

- Eat food with little nutritional value

- Don't exercise

- Avoid feeling your feelings

- Believe you have no choice but to work at a job you don't like

- Complain about how all relationships are difficult

- Spend more time observing life (watching television, movies, athletic events, etc.), than living life

- Defend adamantly how you are right and everyone else is wrong

- Avoid participating in any kind of religious or spiritual practice

In order to remain in denial, you have to block out all positive forces, both from without and from within, that are pushing you forward into awareness. Skepticism keeps denial in place. So does sarcasm. Personal growth is a strong developmental force. It takes a lot of energy to resist and stay in denial.

Kim had a difficult childhood. Kim was ten years old when her parents divorced after a stormy relationship. Kim quickly lost faith in the goodness of life and became an angry child. She overate and withdrew from social activities, preferring the television to real friendships.

By the time she was a teenager, she had become a hardened cynic. Unfortunately, it wasn't just a developmental stage. Her outlook on life was "be careful or someone will get you, so always do what you can to get them first!" That attitude was successful in keeping people away from her. Kim was as prickly as a cactus! Even though she was very intelligent, Kim had trouble keeping a job. A few supervisors were brave enough to attempt to talk to her about her attitude, but Kim was able to ignore them, too, by rationalizing that they simply didn't like her. She was right, of course. Because she was so steeped in her own defensive anger, it was hard for anyone to like her. You could see her anger on her face, in the way she walked, and how quickly she exploded at anything that upset her.

Kim had one friend who was very much like her. Kim and Pat got along well because they shared the same negative worldview—that is, until Pat began to change. Pat was diagnosed with a stress-related illness and began therapy to reduce her resentful response to life that was irritating her immune system. As Pat began to realize the price she was paying for her negativity, she started learning how to make other mental and emotional choices besides anger. Pat was moving into *awareness*, the second level of transformation.

Kim, frightened of losing her one friend, doubted that Pat's changes would hold. When Pat acted more patient in a situation where she would formerly have been belligerent, Kim would say sarcastically, "Fine, but let's see if you're still handling this the same way next week!"

Kim felt a need to deny Pat's personal growth in order to protect herself from the dangerous possibility that Pat might grow beyond her. Of course, if Pat could change, so could Kim. But Kim so identified herself with her own angry, difficult personality that she was afraid of who she would be without it.

Awareness often comes when someone close to us changes his or her life for the better. Eventually, their improvement is evident to everyone around them. To those in denial, it is as if their closed eyes have now been opened at least a crack.

During the next six months, Kim watched as Pat slowly began to enjoy her life more and more. Pat lost weight, softened her harsh judgments, and even began dating! Kim was surprised that Pat didn't waver in her progress.

Awareness is a little pinpoint of light that lets us know there *is* hope at the end of the tunnel. That's important, because when hope begins to enter the picture, powerlessness (which is one of the main components of denial) begins to dim.

Kim eventually began modeling her own behavior after her friend Pat's, except that she didn't go to therapy. She was sure she didn't need anyone telling her what to do! But she did go to Weight Watchers® and she even attempted to refrain from judging the other people she met there. *Maybe they aren't all jerks*, she said to herself. She also tried to curb her impulse to curse at all the stupid drivers on the road who made her angry.

We'll get back to Kim and Pat in a moment, but first let's review the first stage of the Levels of Transformation. The first level (which is also the heaviest and most restrictive) is *denial*. In the denial stage, you feel like a victim, hopeless, powerless, and resistant to change your life in any way for the better. One "advantage" of denial is that you don't have to try to change because you don't believe change is possible. Also, you have no responsibility because you are always the victim. Skepticism and sarcasm are major tools you can use to help you remain in denial. After all, if there is no hope, there is no future in trying to change.

The second stage of the Levels of Transformation is *awareness*, and it is one step up from denial. Observing someone else make successful changes in their life often plants the seed of awareness. When you begin to entertain the possibility of change, there is a rush of positive energy that is released mentally, emotionally, and physically. Hope is a major factor of inspiration!

There are some peculiarities of awareness that need to be mentioned. As soon as you come out of your own denial, you will have the uncanny ability to notice other people in denial! You may even experience an overwhelming urge to tell them all about what you see them doing that isn't working for them. Such information, no matter how well-intentioned it may be, is seldom appreciated. So in order to move forward into an increased awareness yourself, it is best that you concentrate your focus on just yourself.

Once you experience the empowering hope of change, you may suddenly feel as though you are no longer a victim. While that's a wonderful feeling, it's not entirely true. What you are now is an aware victim. Being aware of what you are doing and changing your behavior are two distinctly different things. Because the seed of awareness has just been planted, it must be nourished carefully or it will not grow.

Most people set themselves up for disappointment by expecting too much from themselves after first experiencing awareness. Exercising every day of the week or avoiding all desserts forever are unrealistic beginning goals that will prove too hard to meet. Then when you can't do it perfectly, you blame yourself instead of the unnecessarily ambitious goals you had set. To best navigate the sea of awareness, start small and don't increase your goals until you have successfully maintained the first goal for at least a month. Let's check back with Kim and Pat and see how they are doing with their changes.

Pat continued with her therapy, even though Kim made fun of her. In the process, Pat began to uncover some of the more painful reasons she'd been so angry. In that stage of her awareness, Pat began to withdraw from Kim because Kim's negativity and sarcasm were too upsetting for her to handle. Kim, of course, couldn't understand why Pat was retreating from their relationship and, as a result, her feelings were hurt.

In the meantime, Kim used her time away from Pat to try something new. After resisting exercise for so many years, she suddenly discovered that walking briskly for at least thirty minutes a day made her feel better than she could ever remember. One day while on one of her walks, she noticed a mother and daughter strolling along together holding hands. Usually, that kind of tender scene would have made her angry. On that day, however, a profound sadness washed over her, a sadness that she identified with the pain she felt from the loss of her mother's attention when she was a child. For the first time in many years, Kim went home and cried. She wasn't exactly sure why she was crying; but afterwards, she felt much better.

The next day, however, Kim was once again in a bad mood and ended up verbally attacking a coworker for some small infraction at the office. As she had once before, her supervisor called her in and warned her about her attitude at work. This time was different for Kim, for she realized she was out of line and she actually felt frightened about losing her job. Kim also recognized that her behavior that day was simply an extension of a pattern that had plagued her all her life. For the first time, Kim considered the possibility that she needed to learn how to respond differently to people and situations.

The possibility of really being wrong about how she was treating others was a big difference for Kim. That's what awareness is all about—seeing with different eyes. Whereas denial keeps one blind to new possibilities, awareness allows for all kinds of new options to appear.

The next of the Levels of Transformation is *confusion*. Kim's willingness to admit to herself that she needed to change her attitude, not that somebody should change theirs, was a major opening in her life. Options descended from all directions and Kim had trouble sorting them all out. She was considering self-improvement, but what was her next step? She looked on the Internet and discovered a whole world of options and classes she'd never seen before. Then she remembered a memo that had crossed her desk for a training class on communication that would be paid for by her employer. Was it a good idea to go to a company-sponsored class or should she find one where no one knew her? Kim was thoroughly confused!

Confusion is the third step of transformation, and the stage most often overlooked by those who are in the process of changing. Once you become aware of all the possibilities that you had effectively blocked out while in denial, it can be overwhelming to discover just how many choices you actually have! It is then that you realize you have to make your next choice. Most people are both excited and scared with that responsibility. Confusion can also be called fuzzy fear. If you really let yourself know what you are afraid of, you have to do something about it. Therefore, if you don't know what you're afraid of, you can't possibly take any action. The fuzzy fear delays your need to respond and gives you time to sort out your choices.

People often ask us how long this confusion lasts. Sorry, but there's no exact answer to that question. However, if you're still confused two years from now, that's definitely too long. You may be clinging to confusion in order to avoid making a difficult decision. You also may be holding on to a possibility that you have no real intention of carrying through.

If you find that confusion is a regular and major component of your life, that's another matter altogether. Living every day in confusion is more than just moving through the Levels of Transformation. Perpetual difficulty in making decisions or in prolonged procrastination as a way of life warrants a visit to a professional to look more deeply at the psychological and possibly organic reasons you continue to be confused.

Confusion, as we are discussing it in this model of the Levels of Transformation, is a natural step of experience as we open up to being responsible human beings making the best choices we can at the time.

It can be a difficult time. You are now more aware of what you want, but remain confused about what choices to make in order to go about getting what you want. This is the stage when you can't decide what to wear or where to go for dinner or what to eat when you get there. Everything seems to be more of an effort than ever before. Here are some tips to help you deal with the confusion:

- Don't fight it, it only makes things worse.

- Ask yourself what it is that you're pretending not to know.

- At a gentle pace, gather information to give you more clarity.

- Don't get compulsive about gathering information.

- Stay on one possibility before you look at another.

- Ask others how they worked through similar choices.

- Trust that you will wake up one day and the confusion, like the fog, will have lifted.

- Give yourself a reasonable deadline before taking another step if the confusion hasn't lifted.

After a few weeks of confusion, Kim contacted Pat and shared with her that she was actually thinking of taking a personal growth class on communication because she realized she was unable to control her anger at work. She also complimented Pat on her new changes and even admitted that she had been jealous of her friend's amazing progress.

Pat softened and agreed to meet Kim and tell her about what she'd experienced with her own changes. Kim felt better immediately. She really valued her friendship with Pat and was eager to feel better about herself. Pat told Kim all about her work with her therapist and encouraged Kim to take one of the classes she was considering. They talked about the pros and cons of her options and even though Kim was still nervous, she was determined to take the next step.

Integration is the next rung on the Levels of Transformation. It is often depicted in comic strips as a light bulb above someone's head as the symbol for a new idea. We do know of some cases where people have had a sudden epiphany that they have remembered forever. Most of the people we've worked with, however, find integration as a quiet change that appears in the middle of the night with little or no fanfare.

A common example of moving through the Levels of Transformation to integration is how you feel when you begin a new job. No matter how much you thought you knew before you arrived, the first few days make it seem as though you don't know a thing. You are in *denial*. A few days later, however, you can actually find your way to the copy machine by yourself, answer your complicated phone system, and maybe even use your computer for a few things. You are now in *awareness*. Just when you are beginning to feel competent, you are asked to do something that is totally confusing. You have to ask questions that show you don't fully understand the task. And then one morning you come to work and just do your job. It all seems to flow. You know what to do, when to do it, and you are busy doing it. That's *integration*. You probably didn't look at your watch and say, "Wow, it's ten o'clock on Thursday and I am in integration at work!"

This is the way most people experience moving into integration. It is a subtle experience that often gets missed as a point of reference, and yet it is critical to one's sense of competence and personal growth.

Integration is important, because at this point you no longer feel like a victim. All your confused fears of responsibility have lifted and you are just responsible. And it feels good! It's just plain easier to be responsible than it is to worry about it. When you have moved into integration, you have a marked increase of self-confidence and self-determination. You feel as though you have the power to move forward in your life. Of course, you may still have times of doubts and concerns; but those times don't last as long as they used to. You now possess the confidence to work through your challenges more quickly.

Kim checked out several class options and picked the one she felt most directly addressed her needs. Just showing up for the first class was a positive achievement. Her teacher explained to the class that if they were really committed to improving their communications, they would no doubt learn things about themselves that they would find uncomfortable. Not only was Kim committed, she was determined to improve her ability to deal more effectively with others. These attitudes were strong indicators of her move into integration.

You might think that the Levels of Transformation model ends with integration. Granted, integration is a major step up from denial, but there are still two more levels before it is complete.

New feelings is the level beyond integration. With the confidence gained from integration, it is natural for the fears that have controlled you to dissipate, allowing you to feel differently about challenges that you previously found frightening.

In Kim's case, it was joining a gym. She had always made fun of the "stupid people" who worked out at the gym with all those machines. Then one day, that exercise equipment didn't look so stupid after all. Kim was experiencing new feelings about an old subject. By that time, she had been walking for several months, so exercise had become a regular part of her life. Her involvement with Weight Watchers was gradually producing results and she was losing weight at a slow but steady pace. For the first time in her life, she wanted to move her body even more!

She had heard that the gym in her neighborhood offered yoga and dance classes. Kim was admittedly astounded at herself for even considering joining. Her new feelings meant that her lifelong resistance to change had begun to crack. With her new-found confidence, Kim joined the gym. She was happier than she had been her entire adult life.

Another example of the "new feelings" stage are those people who have had a lifetime of difficulties in maintaining successful intimate relationships who are suddenly willing to risk getting married. If they have gone through the Levels of Transformation, they are willing to risk matrimony because their old negative thoughts and feelings are no longer blocking their ability to feel lovable and, therefore, to love some-one else.

When you are in this stage of new feelings, it is amazing to look back at your life. Don't be surprised if you find it hard to believe the way you led your life when you were in denial.

The last Level of Transformation is *new behavior*. At this point, you not only feel responsible, you are responsible. You know in a deep and immutable way that you can handle whatever comes your way. If you are at a party and are offered your favorite food (the one in which you used to overindulge), you will be able to taste it, enjoy it, and have no fear of overeating. Or if you have been a workaholic, you will be able to leave the office at the same time as everyone else without feeling guilty, and you will be able to go home and enjoy your evening. If you couldn't get off the couch to exercise before, you now find that you're dedicated to your new daily exercise routine and that you don't feel as good if you happen to miss a workout. The desire to take care of yourself seems natural, not forced.

The media will try to convince you that you can glide easily out of denial and move immediately into new behavior *if* you'll just buy their latest and greatest product. That is simply not true. The process moves gradually but steadily through all the emotional physical stages we've described—mental, emotional, and ultimately physical. And we must move through each of those stages if we truly want to make lasting changes. When you attempt to jump directly from denial to new behavior, you haven't established the internal structure necessary to maintain your new choices over the long haul. Think back over your own life. How many times have you tried to make that leap and been disappointed?

How long does all this take? It varies, of course, from one individual to another. It also depends on what it is you are choosing to change. You can be in different stages at the same time with the various issues of your life. You could be in *new behavior* with your career choice and be in *denial* in how you feel about your body. You could be in *confusion* about romantic relationships and be in *integration* about your physical health.

The more areas of your life you move from *denial* to *new behavior*, however, the more congruent your whole life will become. Eventually, you will find that you prefer working and socializing with people who are on their own paths of transformation. In fact, you may find that visiting your old friends or relatives who are still in the *denial* phase isn't much fun. You may be surprised to discover that you don't have much to talk about after the first few minutes. At that point, you have to make a choice. Do you value the relationship enough to continue as it has been? Or do you wish to limit how much time you spend with that person? Be careful, however. Judging that person for being where they are is not a thought in keeping with your *awareness* stage. After all, you were once there yourself. You know from your own personal experience that there were a variety of events in your life that had to occur before you were eventually able to make the decision to escape from *denial* and move into the stage of *awareness*. Appreciating someone where they are, without trying to change them, is one of the hardest yet highest acts of human love.

So, what happened to Kim as she moved into *new behavior*? She not only took that first communication class, but continued through several more advanced courses as well. She applied what she learned to her job, to her personal relationships, and to herself. Kim began to ask herself what she really wanted to do now that she'd actually grown up. When she was really honest with herself, she realized her current job no longer had any appeal. She eventually became a fitness instructor! She was particularly good at helping motivate people who hated exercise, because she could relate to all their fears and excuses. Sometimes, she even told them her personal story, which almost always inspired them to stay in their program. If you were to see snapshots of Kim—one when she was in *denial* and another when she was in her *new behavior*—you would find it hard to believe it was the same person. In addition to the changes in her body, the look on her face is so different you would hardly recognize her. Kim moved from being an unhappy young woman who felt victimized by the world to a strong, in-charge woman who's taken control of her life. And you know what? If Kim can do it, so can you!

While we said the last of the Levels of Transformation was *new behavior*, the truth is that the transformation continues. It continues because once you are in *new behavior*, you will forever be discovering new things you want to learn, challenge, and accomplish. You'll never go back into *denial*. You may visit denial at some time, but you can no longer live there once you have become truly aware. It is common for people to move back and forth between *awareness* and *confusion* before stepping across the invisible line into *integration*. And *integration* can last a long time before *new feelings* and ultimately *new behaviors* make their appearance. So, be patient with yourself. In the next chapter you will learn how to stay self-connected as you move along the path of transformation.

13

Getting to Your Center

Once you've progressed through all the Levels of Transformation, you'll have the consciousness necessary to maintain your new behavior. Even if you momentarily forget what you've learned and how your body feels, you can always return to the new behavior. In times of stress, you may revert to old habits. The difference now is that you won't be in denial about what you're doing, and you'll be able to move out of that old behavior with greater ease and in a shorter period of time than in the past.

Linda's mother and father died within four months of one another. "I found myself deep in grief. My body felt like it was made of lead and I slept a tremendous amount. My exercise program went by the wayside. I was determined to stay with the grieving process, however, as it had been my habit over the years to gloss over sadness and keep myself busy in order not to feel."

During that emotional time, Linda says that she overindulged in her comfort foods and, as a result, gained weight. "I knew exactly what I was doing," admits Linda. "It was not unconscious eating. The difference from my old behavior was that I didn't berate myself for overeating or not exercising. I was gentle to myself. After all, how often do both of your parents die in just a matter of months?"

Linda's innermost vulnerable self was feeling intensely sad and abandoned. She says that what she didn't need at that time was an inner
critical parent getting on her case. So the nurturing adult within her
was kind to her inner child. But still, she didn't use this as an excuse to
go on a binge and use this sad circumstance to redefine her life and her
eating patterns for years to come.

"I observed my old eating habits while I went through the grieving
process, and I did so without self-criticism or guilt. As I began to move
through the deepest part of the grief, my desire for comfort food began
to diminish and I began to miss my workouts. I resumed walking and I
eventually went back to the gym. Without really concentrating on it, I
soon lost all the weight I had gained."

Everyone has within them a deep, quiet place where they feel safety
and peace. The physical placement of that center varies with the individual. Many Eastern traditions and martial art practitioners talk about
this center as the "haufa" or "dantian," and suggest that it exists about
two inches below the belly button. Some people in the West believe the
center of their body is in their solar plexus, others in their heart. "During my grieving process," Linda says, "I spent as much time as possible
getting to my center."

When you locate this quiet and peaceful place inside you, it's like
finding a hidden treasure! To do so is a major step on your path to
becoming balanced emotionally, physically, mentally, and spiritually.
Linda says people often have no idea what she's talking about when she
speaks of this inner center of tranquility and safety. If you, too, are puzzled, don't be alarmed. We'll explain it to you as best we can.

There are four categories most people fall into when experiencing
their center. The first is utilized by those who have been meditating for
years and who know exactly what that center feeling is and how to
access it at will. They are dedicated to spending as much time as possible in that centered feeling and sometimes resent having to come out of
that state of consciousness and back into the outer world. If this
describes you, your challenge is not so much how to find your center,

but rather how to live consciously from that center with your eyes open on a day-to-day basis.

The second are individuals who realize that they may be spending more time feeling "centered" than they would have guessed. Without calling it "being centered," they may have always had a natural inclination to go into nature when feeling stressed, or otherwise know how to "zone out" without using drugs, alcohol, food, television, or the computer. They know how to easily balance themselves. In other words, they are already practicing "being centered" without calling it that. These people also identify with other common ways of finding balance:

- When thinking of the past or future, they make a point of bringing their thoughts into the present.

- They observe and appreciate beauty in all things—nature, babies, animals, people, etc.

- When listening to music, they become joyfully lost in the melody and rhythm.

- They dance and they sing.

- They appreciate and participate in all kinds of creativity.

- They know how to play.

- They are instinctively and genuinely grateful for life.

- They know how to enjoy being quiet by themselves.

The third group is made up of people for whom it has been so long since they felt relaxed, safe, and peaceful that they can barely remember the feeling. In the meantime, they have come to rely on food or some other substance as a means to blocking their anxiety. The last time they felt truly relaxed, safe, and peaceful all at the same time may have been when they were a child. While their memories of those times may have dimmed, their bodies remember. Their bodies are also quite aware of when they're *not* experiencing those wonderful feelings.

When you were a child, time stretched out in front of you like a never-ending road. You could play for hours on end, totally self-absorbed. Do you remember what you liked to play as a kid? Can you recall being so wrapped up in that activity that you had no sense of time passing? Did you ever just lie under a tree and watch the branches gently move with the wind? Think back to what your peaceful moments were like when you were young. Most of them will be simple. Children often have more fun with the box than the toy that came in it. The ability to see the world as wondrous keeps the experience of living exciting. Being outside under the stars was once a magical time, wasn't it? When was the last time you danced in the light of the moon?

Begin to notice children. Watch them and let their actions and imagination lead you to your own. Try coloring a picture or finger painting or riding a bike. Notice how your body feels when you do these things! If you have a tendency to feel embarrassed when doing something new or different, you may have to try each one several times to get to the true pleasure and peace they can offer you.

The fourth group of people has no mental or physical memory of ever feeling safe, relaxed, or peaceful. They struggle every day just to survive. Their childhood was so fraught with fear and every kind of abuse imaginable that they remain hyper-vigilant, fully expecting the worst to happen at any moment. These are people who are likely to be high achievers, often denying their anxiety and fear by learning, doing, and striving to be the best. However, no matter what they do, it's not ever good enough in their eyes. Or on the other end of the spectrum, they may have trouble staying on purpose and achieving anything on a regular basis.

They can almost always benefit from professional therapy to help them identify and then heal those early childhood wounds, to help them learn how to see their current world as safe, and to help them modify their overactive habitual response to stress. It is not uncommon to find that individuals with eating disorders were abused in their younger years, even if they have no conscious memory of that experience. Their extra pounds insulate them from being hurt again. If you feel like you may be one of those people in this fourth group and you have a problem with food as your substance, you are a good candidate for professional therapy.

It would be wonderful if we could all heal ourselves. But like a surgeon trying to operate on himself, it just doesn't work. If you have had a poor experience with therapy in the past, please don't give up. Interview several therapists until you find one with whom you have some rapport. If you're someone who doesn't trust easily or if you find yourself in the fourth group described above, it is unreasonable to expect to find a therapist whom you immediately trust one hundred percent.

But once you rebuild that bridge of trust with one person, the flow of positive life energy can run back and forth with ease, as it was intended to do in the first place. Getting to your center begins with discovering that you can trust yourself, your world, and a higher power. While you're working on these major tasks here are some ways to practice getting to your center.

- Stop doing and simply relax. Continue to do nothing but enjoy your surroundings for at least ten minutes.

- Breathe deeply, inhaling all the way down and allowing the air to fill your lower lungs and forcing your belly to rise. Exhale slowly, letting all that air out in a slow steady stream. Notice how your shoulders move up and down when you breathe like that? Imagine that with each breath you are releasing tension from every part of your body.

- If you don't already have one already, create a safe place in your house where you can go to feel relaxed and peaceful. Notice what inspires safety—a soft blanket, a pillow, a candle, or some other object you enjoy are a just few suggestions. Practice going to that place and breathe deeply, as suggested in the paragraph above. Be present in that moment and allow the feeling of safety to surround you, inside and out.

- Remember some of your favorite places that you've visited or where you've always wanted to go. As you sit in your safe place, imagine being in one of those favorite locations. See it, feel it, hear it, touch it. Allow yourself to go deeper into this fantasy and relax even more. Experience in your mind how it is to feel safe.

- As you practice finding a variety of ways to get to your center, make a note of them so you can use them in different situations. It is handy to be able to sit in an airport when delayed, for example, and use this simple and easy method to relax.

Too often, adults use overeating in an attempt to experience that peaceful and safe feeling at their center. In filling themselves up, they hope to feel fulfilled. What happens instead is they end up feeling bloated, uncomfortable, and guilty.

During the time her parents were ill and eventually died, Linda practiced a variety of ways of getting to her center. When you are in grief or trauma, the need to be centered is paramount. When emotional, however, it can be very difficult to find your balance, let alone your center! Linda recalls the day her father died. "My husband and I drove to the closest beach, a hundred miles from where we lived. Somehow, the sound of the ocean's waves crashing on the shore felt comforting. As I sat on the sand and felt the rhythmic flow of that huge body of water, I began to find my center. I was still lightly aware of my grief, but I was also in my center."

Just a few months later when her mother died, Linda was on a business trip in Houston, Texas. "That day, I walked slowly for hours down a beautiful path by a river, just observing nature and the flow of life represented in the steady movement of the water. Again, I had found my center. I also meditated, cried, got support from loved ones, and wrote in my journal."

Nature is obviously one of Linda's favorite ways to feel centered. Mountains, forests, lakes, fields, deserts, or your own backyard may be what calms and relaxes you. "Recognizing the experiences that help you find your center in advance of tough times is an advantage," says Linda.

"Then when the difficult times come along, you can physically go to that location, as I did when I went to the beach." If it's impossible to physically go to your favorite location, you can always go there in your mind through visualization.

Becky

When Becky first came to see Linda for therapy, she could hardly sit still. Words shot out of her mouth in rapid-fire succession as she told Linda why she'd decided to see her. As she spoke, Becky kicked her foot back and forth. Every cell in her body seemed to be in perpetual motion. At first, Becky was very resistant to any kind of meditation or even relaxation.

Surprisingly, she readily admitted that the reason she was so busy was to avoid her feelings. If she sat still for too long, she said, she would usually begin to cry. Unfortunately, she'd been continuously busy for the last five years and even though she was only twenty-seven years old, she was exhausted. She believed that caffeine and all the extra attention she paid to her work were her salvation.

No wonder she resisted slowing down and quieting her mind! Her emotions were right there just waiting for the opportunity to be expressed. After a few sessions with Linda, Becky began to understand the physical and emotional consequences of avoiding her feelings. Although admittedly reluctant, she said she was willing to try to break the pattern.

"We decided she should start small," Linda reports. "Becky began sitting quietly for five minutes early in the morning, not long after she got up and before she started getting ready for work. She discovered this worked best for her."

For two months, Becky continued practicing that routine—five minutes a day in the early morning, just sitting and relaxing. Then the time was expanded to ten minutes, and Becky began to close her eyes and practice focusing her attention on her gentle breathing. As soon as the time was extended to ten minutes, however, Becky began getting emotional. She found herself crying, and not knowing why. However,

Linda had prepared her for that eventuality, and so Becky just let herself cry. Many times, what lies between you and your center are unexpressed emotions.

After getting used to her emotions in small increments, Becky was eventually able to cry at times other than during her quiet relaxation routine. That was an indication that her emotions didn't always have to seep out every time she stopped moving for ten minutes. She remained diligent in her practice and eventually was able to sit still and relax for as long as thirty minutes. This simple method of finding her center slowly but surely had a positive impact upon every aspect of her life.

Linda says that as time went by, she saw less and less of Becky, for her client was now spending more time discovering the world outside of her job. She quit drinking caffeine, began taking a class in meditation, and learned to line dance!

Becky still has more energy than the average person. However, she has learned to balance her activities with rest, relaxation, and fun, instead of focusing entirely on her work. Linda says that when she first met her, Becky was convinced that caffeine and her work were attempts to avoid her emotions, although neither the coffee nor her job fed her emotionally or physically. Now when she finds herself occasionally falling back into that old habit of doing too much, she is able to catch herself in the act, find her center, and successfully interrupt the pattern.

When it comes to making long-term changes, learning new ways to deal with yourself allows new behavior to be a preferred way of living. When you go to the center of your being and actually feel safe and peaceful and relaxed, there is no need to seek elsewhere for those feelings. It is a place that you can count on every moment of every day. The best part is that it's been there all along, right inside your very being! However, the food you choose to eat has a profound effect upon your ability to stay in your center.

14

What Are We Eating
and
How Does It Make Us Feel?

When we are committed to making long-term changes and learning new thoughts and behaviors, another way of finding support is to find out what we are eating and paying attention to how it makes us feel. Most of us are not aware of what we put in our mouths on a daily basis. Neither are we aware of our body's signals. Most importantly, we are not aware of all the negative thoughts we have about ourselves in relationship to our body. Often, we have given up on trying to eat a healthy diet because we've given up hoping that we will ever feel healthy or look good.

The fact is, we are all born beautiful creatures and part of the Divine. Have you ever stopped to reflect on this? You don't have to look a certain way for this to be true; it just Is. You don't have to be healthy for this to be true; it just Is. You are beautiful! And as we said earlier, you are programmed for joy, happiness, and bliss—even in relationship to your health, the food you eat, and your looks. So what is it that keeps us feeling hopeless instead of feeling bliss?

Think of the Source of the Divine as water coming out of a garden hose. When you are young, you freely play in the water and never question if there will be enough water. You simply have fun spraying your-self and plants and others with this abundant water. You feel connected to it and you believe that it will never run dry. As you grow older, you start hearing such things as "don't do that," "you should do this," "you look like this," and "your dreams are stupid, if not impossible." With this input, you slowly form beliefs about yourself and soon your once flowing garden hose, the one that kept you in touch with your inner wisdom, now seems kinked. You no longer believe there is enough life vitality available from the Source because now only a trickle of water is coming out. You feel disconnected and do not trust the Source to give you water or guidance. These beliefs eventually become what we project outward as ourselves, even though we are so much more.

Our beliefs are at the foundation of our thinking, and our thinking is the foundation of our behaviors. Our feelings are the guide that lets us know what we are thinking and therefore what we really believe. For example, if you believe you are unlovable and ugly and are undisci-plined, then that is what your actions will portray. In reality, you are still that beautiful, blissful person you were when you were born.

So how do we get back to the bliss? We've given you several exercises to help you get in touch with your feelings. Your feelings are your guid-ance system that will point the way to your thinking and it is your thinking that will point the way to your beliefs that may be blocking the path to your blissful state and your flow from the Source.

Keeping a Food Journal

Would you like a simple, surefire way to uncover your beliefs about yourself? Start keeping a food journal, because keeping track of your eating patterns will reveal what you really believe about yourself. Take the time every day to honor yourself by writing down *everything* you put into your mouth. The practice of keeping a daily food journal will start you on a path of becoming aware not only of what you're eating, but why. It will help show you what you are feeling, thinking, and believing about yourself. By keeping a daily food journal, you will slowly begin to hear your inner wisdom and gain access to your most important God-like self. Such access will bring you into alignment with your bliss. And we all want to experience bliss.

Kathleen's own story illustrates clearly the benefits of keeping such a food journal. She admits to having resisted the idea for some time. She realizes now that resistance should have been the first clue that she needed to do it. When she finally got started, she says a whole new world opened up for her. "What I quickly discovered," she says, "is that I found out that I was eating a lot more chocolate than I thought I was. It had become my lover, my companion. It was sweet, reliable, easily available, and it made me feel good." Kathleen says she soon realized that she was eating chocolate at times when she felt disconnected from the ones she loved.

"I began thinking about my childhood. I was the oldest of thirteen children. I was 'Miss Responsibility' and took care of my siblings. I did everything well or not at all. What I lacked was a sense of connection to my family. I didn't have a feeling of belonging, only of being needed. Early on, I formed a belief that my only worth was in filling the needs of others, even if it meant abandoning myself. I lost myself. Over the years, I tried to fill this gaping hole with chocolate."

Kathleen continued to record what she ate and how it made her feel. As she did so, all those long-suppressed feelings from her childhood started bubbling up and spilling themselves across the pages of her journal—anger, loneliness, and fear. In time, she felt liberated from the past that she had stored in every cell of her body and that kept her blocked from her Source.

"I was finally free to make new choices and take responsibility for my own life and what I wanted. After documenting the connection between my emotions and my eating habits, I decided that what I wanted more than anything else was a healthy body and a passion for living. I was determined to break free of the habits created by past emotions. And I have no qualms about saying that chocolate is still one of my favorite foods! I still allow it to give me pleasure; except now I realize that it's a gift I can choose to give myself."

Kathleen says when she does eat chocolate, the messages her body gives her are unmistakable. "When I can eat it and feel my bliss and walk away, I know that everything within me is in harmony. When I have devoured an entire candy bar and don't remember eating it, the message is loud and clear that something in my life is out of balance and I'd better do something about it. It is a signal that I need to go to my feelings and inner wisdom and start writing until I know what is wrong." Kathleen says that, with practice, she is now able to find her way quickly back to her center, to her bliss. "My favorite imagery of that centered feeling is that of a playful child running and skipping through a lawn sprinkler on a warm summer afternoon, knowing I am connected to my Source of life."

So how do you get started? The great thing about keeping a food journal is there's really nothing to it. You only need a few things: a journal (as simple as a notepad or as elaborate as a hardbound book with blank pages), a pen, and a commitment to honor yourself by making at least one journal entry a day, recording all you ate and drank and how you felt during those twenty-four hours.

If you find yourself forgetting to do this every day or if you simply find it too hard, this may be a message that you may not believe yourself worthy of being honored. What do you do when this happens? Write it down! Start your daily entry with: "I do not want to do this," and then write down the reasons why. Remember, *no one but you is going to read this journal* and those you want to read it. Let whatever comes to mind fall out onto the pages. You will soon discover that it's very freeing and eye-opening as you start to see what you are actually eating and how much and under what circumstances. As a natural part of the process, you'll have memories connected to certain foods float up to your consciousness.

You'll also begin noticing certain sensations that are connected to certain foods. Kathleen says that an example of this is when she eats dairy foods, and especially ice cream. When she does that, she says, "About an hour later, my energy is very low and I wake up the next morning with a scratchy throat and a drippy nose and (sorry to get personal here) constipation." After recognizing that ice cream is obviously not a great food for her, she crossed that off her menu. "I don't feel deprived by not eating ice cream. Quite the contrary, I feel deprived of my health and vitality when I do eat it." Because she was keeping a journal, she was able to keep track of those little nuances, those seemingly inconsequential connections that she never would have noticed otherwise. "I would never have known just how unmistakably clearly my body was signaling me. My body was honoring my commitment to health and vitality by letting me know this food did not offer that for me."

Sherry is another example of someone who used a food journal as a way to get in touch with her beliefs. She had gained a lot of weight over the last couple of years and was becoming more moody and depressed. She wasn't aware of what she was eating or how much, so she decided to start a journal to see exactly what it was that she was doing. Every day, she wrote down what she ate and drank. After some time, she started incorporating into her writing how she felt, too. Sherry soon started to see a pattern. She began to realize that she would frequently grab sugared foods and salty, crunchy snacks during the day in a misguided attempt to combat the negativity in her life. She had in-laws that were constantly telling her (and her three small children!) what a "bad" mother she was. She had married and started having children at a very young age, so she was impressionable and believed their input. She started to believe she really was a "bad" mother. She came to realize that her feelings of inadequacy actually stemmed from much earlier on in her life when she felt she had no worth and was unlovable even as a child. She had been using food to help cover over these devastating beliefs and the feelings they produced.

Sherry knew she had no clue how to heal this belief about herself, so she wisely sought counseling. She continued keeping the journal as she got help with a new, healthy eating and exercise program. She slowly formed new thoughts, new beliefs, and new behaviors. The combination of honoring her body and emotions brought her to new spiritual awareness of who she is. She is now a very vibrant and powerful woman.

Another example is Joseph. He came to Kathleen with end-stage liver cancer, the doctors having given him only three more months to live. Together, Kathleen and Joseph devised a clean eating plan for him, plus a regular schedule of cleansing, especially colon hydrotherapy. With the support of his wife, he did great. His energy returned and he was able to travel and do all the things he wanted to do.

There were still times when he would feel sick and the pain would return. He asked Kathleen if she thought there was anything he could do about it. "I asked him to write out what was going on in his life at the time," Kathleen says. "He liked writing on his computer, so he did that. Time and time again, he realized that when he was upset or worried about something, his symptoms would return." Since Joseph was also writing down what he was eating, it wasn't long before he could see that prior to feeling the nausea and pain, he'd been eating foods that weren't on his eating plan. With time, Kathleen adds, Joseph could identify the foods and the emotions that made him sick and use his illness as a barometer for his overall physical, emotional, and spiritual well-being. Joseph lived an active and full life for four more years!

"I had the privilege and honor of being with him on the day he died," Kathleen says, "and to have been a part of his living life fully and consciously and transitioning in that same way." Kathleen says that she is convinced it was his commitment to live life to the limit and to look fear and death in the face and go beyond it that afforded him such a long and satisfying four years. "He continues to be an inspiration and a gift to me."

Tools for Balanced Living

Once you begin keeping a journal, you'll start to get a true picture of what it is that you're eating, thinking, and feeling. So now that you have this new-found knowledge, how do you begin to make changes? We'll give you some simple things you can do. Remember, it's important that you take things one step at a time. You probably already know from experience that trying to do to many things at once is an almost surefire prescription for failure. Continue doing one step until it becomes a natural, everyday occurrence. This will ensure good results, and good results are a natural incentive to go on to the next step.

Take your time. The emotional issues that surround your eating habits and your feelings about yourself did not happen overnight. Take your time. Your intention is to be healthy and vibrant, not win a race. You will be honoring yourself every day you make even the smallest change for the better. So let's get started.

Oxygen—Breathe! Breathe! And then breathe some more! Your reaction is probably to say, "What's the big deal? I breathe all the time without even thinking about it!" The problem is that many of us have become shallow breathers. Fortunately, this is very easy to change. Before you eat or drink, take three deep breaths. See if you can cause your chest to expand farther each time. Picture your lungs as big bellows that you're filling up with each breath. Oxygen is the food your brain needs to function, so fill up those lungs! You'll need to remind yourself on a regular basis, but eventually you'll get in the habit of deep, healthful breathing.

Water—Drink at least half your body weight in ounces of clean, pure water every day. If you are working out, live in an extremely hot or cold climate, travel, or if you're under stress, pregnant, nursing, smoking, drinking alcohol, or any other situation that puts you out of your normal routine, you need more water. Did you know that when you feel thirsty, you are already "about a quart low?" When you're thirsty, it means you have more free radical damage, more toxins built up in the body, and your electrolytes are out of balance—all because you didn't drink enough water soon enough.

Food—There is no set diet that fits everyone, of course, but there are some general guidelines that do pertain to us all. We'll start by breaking these guidelines down into individual steps. (Again, by taking things one step at a time until they become natural and an everyday occurrence, we increase our chances of success.)

1. Start by eating only those dairy and animal products that are clean (*i.e.,* food that contain no antibiotics, hormones, or other chemicals and additives such as the nitrates commonly found in bacon, lunch meat, and sausage).

2. Next, start to eat only those grains, beans, nuts, seeds, etc., that are free of pesticides and herbicides.

3. Then advance to eating clean fruits and vegetables.

4. Start changing your eating habits so that fruit comprises about ten percent of your diet and vegetables fifty percent. There are a lot of creative cookbooks for preparing vegetables. Have fun finding the ones that appeal to you. Take advantage of the wide range of flavors and colors of vegetables. Each color has different nutrients.

5. Introduce three to four ounces of protein at each meal. Everyone is different. Some people may want soy protein; some may prefer cottage cheese, while others may want a steak. Protein is the building block for every part of your body. When we fail to provide our body with enough protein, it cannot perform its daily functions well and neither can it build healthy new cells.

6. Now start removing all the refined carbohydrates from your daily diet. These are occasional treats, not nourishment! They do not support our goals of health and vitality. Write down in your journal a list of all the refined and chemical-laden foods (diet colas, cookies, cakes, pies, donuts, white rice, white pasta, white bread, sugared cereals, etc.) in your diet. Don't lie to yourself. Write them all down. Kathleen confesses, "I felt pretty pitiful when I wrote my list out. But I realized I couldn't change if I did not know what it was I was putting into my body." In your journal, write your intention and then the steps

you will take to eliminate these foods from your diet. Take it in steps, eliminating one thing at a time. This is the point at which emotions will start flooding the pages of your journal. Why? Because these refined-carbohydrate concoctions have become the comfort foods of our society. They give us a temporary high that makes us feel good about ourselves. How can you deal with your beliefs about yourself without the comfort food? Go back and repeat the three-step exercise in Chapter Three ("Coming Down from the Moon Palace"). This will help you reconnect to your inner wisdom and your own personal place of safety.

7. To help put it all together, start with clean food and water, then picture your plate at each meal. Vegetables comprise fifty to sixty percent of what you have on that plate, thirty to forty percent of what's on your plate is protein, and the rest are complex carbohydrates. For example, say you had a small chicken breast on your plate along with one-half cup of cooked green beans and some cooked zucchini and tomatoes. Or you could have a salad of mixed greens and cut-up vegetables with some olive oil and vinegar dressing. Or perhaps you have two to three scrambled eggs with cut-up sautéed vegetables and a piece of fruit. Or a tofu and vegetable stir-fry with a half-cup of brown rice and a mixed green salad. Are you starting to get the picture? By visualizing before each meal what you're going to put on your plate, you will have a greater awareness and better control over what you eat. By thinking about it beforehand, you will be consciously choosing what you eat instead of just eating from an unconscious emotional place. This is a powerful position to be in.

8. Take time to honor yourself by making food-planning part of your weekly schedule. How many lists of chores and errands do you use in an average week? Too often, however, we tend to forget the most important task of all—how we should nourish

ourselves. Once a week, sit down, have a drink of water, and think through the coming week. What will you need in regards to food? Are there times when you'll be on the road? Are there activities after work that will require you to eat quick meals? Make a grocery list based on what your needs will be. Eat a delicious meal first and *then* go grocery shopping. (It helps to keep your budget and waistline stable if you are not shopping on an empty stomach.) When you get home from the grocery store, wash all the fruits and vegetables. Cut up the vegetables and store them in containers. This makes them easy to grab and use even in those harried times. Bake that chicken; make that tuna or tofu salad or whatever you have so that it's ready to eat when you are. By doing all this, you have honored yourself and your family (and besides, you're now prepared for the entire week and will eliminate any excuses you might have made for not eating healthy!).

Exercise—Do something to get your body moving every day. If you are not used to any physical exertion, start small. There are lots of things you can do to get started. For instance, park your car farther away from the door so you at least have to walk a couple of times a day. Go up and down the stairs at work or home a couple of times a day while talking on your cordless phone. Get up from your desk at work or your recliner at home every hour, take a deep breath, just jump in place for a minute or two, and then stretch. After you get home from work, have your walking shoes in the car and put them on and walk around your block *before* you go into the house. Get creative! Find little ways to move your body.

Here are some other ideas to help you get started on changing the way you live:

- Get adequate sleep and down time. Don't keep pushing to work harder and longer. Listen to your body. If you find it difficult to get up in the morning, your body is telling you something. Your body needs this down time in order to repair and rebuild itself. Without it, you are going to be running on an empty tank.

- Prayer and meditation have proven to be beneficial in improving overall health. They center and balance the body while at the same time helping you to connect to your inner wisdom, the very source of life. A powerful prayer or meditation is to just focus on all for which you are thankful.

- Think positive thoughts. Never underestimate the power of positive thinking. Thoughts are powerful because they create the beliefs by which you live. Bless your life. Use positive affirmations. Author Louise L. Hay has done a remarkable job in teaching people how to use affirmations, and in her book, *You Can Heal Your Life*, she gives many examples and stories.

This may seem like a long laundry list of things to do. We agree. It *is* a long list. But as we've said before, you are to take things one step at a time. As you practice and incorporate each step into your routine, it will become a natural part of the flow of your everyday life.

As you progress, it is important with each new step to continue recording in your journal your activities, the food you eat, and your thoughts. Write out each new intention and the steps you will be taking to realize this intention. Commit to at least one journal entry a day. Remember, this is a journey and not a race. And at all times, be truthful to yourself in your journal. You cannot create the life you want if you are lying and hiding from any negative beliefs you may have about yourself. Let whatever comes up spread itself onto the pages. This is a powerful exercise. It helps you stay focused on honoring yourself.

Kathleen recently had the honor of hearing Dr. Michael Beckwith speak. Dr. Beckwith is the founder of Agape, a large multicultural church, and a powerful man who walks his talk. He told this wonderful story of an older, retired gentleman who went into an antique store and was admiring a particularly beautiful piece of furniture. The shopkeeper had seen the old man in the shop before and each time he would always look around and then end up admiring that same piece of furniture. One day, the old man said he wanted to buy the piece, but asked if could put it away in layaway, as he could not afford to pay for it outright. The shopkeeper agreed, but doubted that the old man would live to pay it off. Every month, the old gentleman would come in to admire the piece and make another payment. After a couple of years, he'd finally paid it off and it was his. The shopkeeper said to the old man, "I know it's none of my business, but why did you want that piece of furniture? I can see that you are old and it was obviously not easy for you to pay for it." The old man said, "I live in only one room, but it is my home. And I only allow the best in my home." The old man is an example to us.

Your body is your earthly home. Shouldn't you only put the very best into it? Similarly, aren't our minds the instrument with which we create? Shouldn't we give our minds only the best thoughts? Likewise, our spirit is our connection to the source of all life and health, therefore should we not give it the time and nourishment it needs so that we can be the best? With deserved attention and effort on our part, we can be who we were created to be.

15

Removing Caffeine and Aspartame from Your Diet

You have taken steps to get to your center and journal what you are eating and feeling. You are making lifestyle changes that are supporting life. Congratulations! By choosing to read this chapter, you are taking a major step toward having a vital life instead of depleting it. The withdrawal from the addictive substances caffeine and aspartame (the chemical most commonly used a sugar substitute in diet colas and other drinks and foods) can be challenging, to say the least. We often don't realize that we're using these substances to fill a void in our lives, such as unfulfilling jobs or relationships. Nor do we readily recognize that we might be using them because we're not getting enough sleep or because we're lethargic, when it could be that these symptoms are simply due to a diet that lacks in nutrition. Whatever our reason (or reasons) for using caffeine and aspartame, they deplete our vital life source.

This is a good time to pull out your journal and write yourself a letter. Tell your body why you want to get off whatever addictive substance you might be using. Write down any fears you may have about kicking your addiction. Write down how good you're going to feel once you're on the other side of the withdrawal. Tell yourself in your journal about all the positive things that will open up for you in your life once you're free of the addictive drug.

Keep your journal handy. Every day, record what you're experiencing physically and emotionally, describe the thoughts you had throughout the day. Write about how you slept the night before. After a week, reread your journal notes, and you will start seeing subtle changes that you would have missed had you not been writing on a daily basis.

"Many people ask me in my practice if I think they are addicted to caffeine and/or to aspartame," says Kathleen. "My answer is always the same. Your body will let you know." She suggests doing without the substance for twenty-four hours to see if you experience any withdrawal symptoms. "These are most often headaches, fatigue, inability to concentrate, mild anxiety or depression, cravings, drowsiness, muscle pain or stiffness, or mild nausea," she says. "If you experience any of these symptoms, you are addicted."

Gently Ease Off Addictive Substances

You have two choices when kicking addictions: go cold turkey or take the more gentle, gradual road. Although everyone is different, Kathleen says that most people just give up if they find the withdrawal is too painful. The cold turkey approach usually does not work for most people, whereas the gentle method is easier on your body and creates fewer withdrawal symptoms. Start by getting your journal out again and writing down what your intention is and what your goal is. For example, you might write:

"My intention is to have an alert, healthy, and vibrant body, mind, and spirit. My goal is to remove all caffeine and aspartame from my body."

By doing that, you are now clear with every cell in your body, your spirit, and your mind what it is you are doing. Now set a realistic deadline for being off the substance. This can be whatever your inner wisdom decides it should be, so take the time to listen. Now write this down in your journal:

"I will take _____ months/weeks to remove these substances from my body."

Next, eliminate one-fourth of a cup of coffee or one-fourth of a can or glass of cola every day for the next two weeks. Then eliminate another one-fourth of a cup, can, or glass for another span of time (whatever time you set for yourself). Keep doing this until you are weaned from the substance. As a last step, replace the substance with purified water, herbal tea (hot or cold), or plain seltzer water with a twist of lemon or lime.

Remember to set realistic goals for yourself. Resist the temptation to become competitive with yourself. Remember to love and honor yourself. Constantly remind yourself of your intention and goals. The results are what you are aiming for. You want to be healthy. Never forget that the gift is in the being, not in the doing. Unfortunately, in our culture, frequently it is only the "doing" that is affirmed. In our society, we are valued if we can do, do, do—and do it fast. Always keep in mind that there is value in simply being who you are—a healthy, vibrant, alert, and loving person.

As you go through the process of ridding your body of addictive substances, continue to write in your journal what comes up for you. What body sensations are you experiencing? What feelings and thoughts are you having? Some people experience headaches, fatigue, and aching all over. Others experience feelings of inadequacy and think that they need to try the substance again to give them the buzz to push forward. Some feel as though their bodies need the chemical stimulation to keep them going. Everyone is different.

The fun part of all this is you will learn about parts of yourself that have been controlling your life on a subconscious, hidden level. When this information surfaces, you will then have the opportunity to look at it and use the techniques we've given you to change those beliefs, transforming them to what you really want for your life. This is the process of living a conscious life. Once you get past the fear of seeing your feelings naked and experiencing the body's reaction to withdrawing from the addictive substance, you will begin to enjoy the most incredible and energizing power. That power is the result of your mind listening to and becoming full partners with your body. Now *that's* a high!

Support Your Body During Withdrawal

Continuing to write in your journal and occasionally go back and read what you've written. Doing so will be an ongoing and important guide to supporting your body. Here are some other general things to keep in mind as you go through the process of withdrawal.

- *Water*—Drink plenty of water to help flush the toxic substances out of your body. Increase your normal intake of water (*i.e.,* a quantity of water equal to half your body weight in ounces), by adding at least two more glasses. You will have fewer withdrawal symptoms if you are hydrated properly!

- *Rest*—Adequate rest is so important. If your intention is to have a healthy body, this is an indispensable part of the formula. Your inner wisdom will guide you as to how many hours you need. If you aren't ready to get up in the morning and you feel as though you're dragging all day, you are not getting enough sleep. Whenever the body is "detoxing" from a depleting substance (such as caffeine and aspartame), it will usually want more sleep, because the detoxification process and the rebalancing of the body take place during our sleeping hours.

- *Diet*—This is the time to load up on nutrient-dense foods. Eat more vegetables and fruit and drink fresh-squeezed juices made from organic vegetables and fruit (and not something in a bottle that's been on a shelf for who knows how long). Eat at least three to four ounces of protein at each meal. Protein provides strength, alertness, and the building blocks to help your body make new, healthy cells, and protein is also needed to help drive all the enzyme and hormonal activity in your body. This is a time to give your body a break by staying away from refined foods and sweets. Your body is doing a wonderful job of getting the toxic substances out of your body by going through the withdrawal process and rebuilding new tissue for a healthier you. Don't punish and deplete it with toxic foods deficient in nutrition.

- *Supplements*—It's helpful at all times, but especially as you are ridding your body of addictive substances, to take a multivitamin and mineral supplement. A good B vitamin that has pantothenic acid (a B vitamin) would also be beneficial. The B vitamins assist in adrenal function. The adrenals are drained by the use of substances such as caffeine. In Chapter Seventeen, we provide you with some resources for these supplements.

Todd's story is a good example how this withdrawal/detoxification process works. Todd is a stockbroker whose job is fast-paced and stressful. He had gained weight over the past several years. When he first discussed his diet with Kathleen, he told her he was drinking three to four diet colas a day. (Diet colas contain both caffeine *and* aspartame.) After recording his food intake for one month, he realized he was actually drinking many more a day—more like six to twelve diet colas.

Todd agreed that he would perform the twenty-four hour test to see if he was addicted. He didn't even make it through the morning. He was anxious, he couldn't focus on his work, and he easily became angry with his fellow workers. To top things off, he also had a pounding headache.

Although he was eventually successful, it took Todd four months to slowly wean his body off the diet colas. Writing in his journal throughout the process helped him discover that he'd been using the addictive substances in the diet cola to cover up his fear of appearing inadequate in front of his peers. The caffeine and aspartame combined to make him artificially feel stronger and more confident. They also helped him to stay awake and alert in the high-speed arena in which he had to function every day. He was used to getting about four to five hours of restless sleep a night and needed the high from the chemicals in the diet cola to keep going.

He supported his body with lots of water, diet, rest, and supplements. Skeptical of this process at first, Todd is now on a campaign to see a caffeine- and aspartame-free world. He feels good, has mental clarity, and sleeps like a baby. He has also gotten counseling to help him deal with his underlying self-image issues. Unlike the past, now he rarely gets the colds and flu that go around the office. As an unexpected bonus and without trying, he lost twenty pounds!

16

Cleansing the Body of Toxins

To continue feeling vital and connected to your inner wisdom, another step is cleansing the body of toxins. Cleansing is another journey of discovery, one that will help free you from habits that have kept you trapped in an unhealthy lifestyle. Cleansing rejuvenates the body, mind, and spirit. As you cleanse the body, toxins are released into the blood so that the body can dispose of them. Because unexpressed emotions have been stored in the cells of the body, you may also release pent-up emotions you never knew you had as the toxins are flushed from your body. Therefore, this process gives you the opportunity to deal with the feelings and cleanse them from your body at the same time.

We know this will come as no surprise to you—*it is very important to journal during a cleansing process*! Writing is an excellent way of getting emotions out of the body. As with the other processes we've discussed, writing also helps you keep track of your physical progress during the cleanse. By taking note of the bodily sensations that come up, you will see that these can range from increased energy and clarity of mind to headaches and body aches. As you record what happens to your body and to your emotions, you will become more adept at hearing your inner wisdom speak to you and you will learn how to interpret it. Your inner wisdom is the part of you that never lies and always works to help you attain your highest good. Your inner wisdom is the best part of you to know and to have an intimate relationship with.

Cleansing is a process that can precipitate reactions that come from toxins being released faster than the liver, kidneys, skin, intestines, and lungs can remove them. Symptoms of a cleansing reaction may include nausea, headaches, swelling in the lymph glands, diarrhea, joint pain, lethargy, skin rashes, anxiety, depression, or flu-like symptoms. This is called a healing or correcting crisis. As the toxins are removed from the cells and move into the blood, your body now has to deal with them in a more aggressive manner. The body had learned to be balanced with the toxins in it, and now it is being told to dispose of them and to rebalance without them.

Sound unpleasant? This process will sometimes feel worse before it feels better. Just remember that any discomfort is a signal to you that your body was indeed toxic and needed to be cleansed. Unhealthy lifestyle patterns often lead to very toxic states inside our bodies.

If you want to move into a new lifestyle pattern, it is frequently advantageous to cleanse the body before your start. You wouldn't put new oil in a car without draining out the old, grungy oil first. The cleansing process for your body is the same concept.

If you have an illness or have never gone through a cleansing before, you should first seek the guidance of a knowledgeable health care practitioner to make sure that you have the knowledge and the support you need to go through this process.

A Simple Cleanse

One day a month or at least one day a quarter, set aside some time just for yourself, a quiet time to reflect on your new goals and the feeling you are going to have when you're healthy and vibrant. You won't be answering phones, faxes, or e-mails. You won't be watching TV or movies. You won't be catching up with friends. This is your time to be with the most important person in your life—*you*. Some of us can't relate to the fact that we are the most important person in our life, but where would your loved ones and coworkers be if you were either partially or totally incapacitated from a sickened body? If you don't take care of you, who will? When you think about it, only you can control and be responsible for you. A good starting place is a cleansed body.

Steps for a One-day Cleanse

1. Drink at least ten glasses of lemon water throughout the day. To make the lemon water, squeeze a wedge of fresh organic lemon into each glass of water. Each medium-size lemon is about six wedges. Also, make sure your water is filtered.

2. After rising and drinking some lemon water, eat one or two pieces of organic fruit. For example, cut up an apple and eat one wedge at a time. Take about a half hour to eat the apple. A short while later, peel an orange and eat one section at a time. Savor each bite as you chew it slowly. In this manner, make the fruit last throughout the morning.

3. Continue drinking lemon water until lunch.

4. At noon, have a large organic salad with a small amount (two tablespoons) of olive oil or flaxseed oil mixed with some freshly squeezed lemon as a dressing. The salad should have at least two cups of a mixed variety of leafy green vegetables (no iceberg lettuce, as it lacks any real nutritional value). Add to the salad a cup or more of cut-up vegetables. Make sure you have different vegetables and different colors, for this makes for more nutrients.

5. Continue to drink your lemon water during the day.

6. Do not snack between meals. Just drink your lemon water.

7. For dinner, have a bowl of at least two cups of steamed vegetables. Again, make sure you have a variety of vegetables and colors.

8. Continue to drink your lemon water until bedtime.

9. During the day and evening when you are not eating, it's important to write in your journal. Make at least three journal entries during this day of cleansing. Write whatever comes to mind. Don't judge it, just write it down. Remember, it is your body, your thoughts, your emotions—in other words, it's your inner wisdom that is speaking to you. Your inner wisdom won't lie to you, so just write the pure essence of what comes up during this time. Kathleen says that the first time she did this, one of the things that came up was anger at her body for not being stronger. "I felt as though I were a wimp compared to others," remembers Kathleen. "My body would get tired easily and collapse. I never realized how angry I was with my body until it fell out on the pages of my journal." This was a destructive way of relating to herself and she knew she needed to change her thoughts about her body and be grateful for how well it had supported her through some very difficult times. "It took time and practice," she says, "but I can honestly say I love my body."

10. Take a twenty- to thirty-minute walk in the morning and again in the late afternoon. This helps the blood and lymph systems move, facilitating the release of toxins during the cleanse.

11. Take time to pray or meditate and to just hear yourself think during the day. Getting in touch with your inner wisdom gives creative energies space to rise to the surface and renew your life. As the day progresses and your negative chatter slows down, so does your mind. When that happens, some great new ideas start to bubble up. This is the fun part of the day. However, if this doesn't happen for you, don't get discouraged. It will with time because that creative energy is the essence of who you are. It is always in there. It just needs some space in order to be recognized and heard. For some of us, it has been stuffed down for so long, it will take some time before it feels permission to be active.

12. Take a cleansing bath before going to bed. One simple bath is to take a pound of sea salt and a pound of baking soda and pour them into a very warm tub of water. Soak in the tub until the water is cool. Then take a lukewarm shower and rinse off using a loofa sponge to wipe the released toxins from your skin.

13. Before going to bed, make another journal entry. How did your day go? How did you feel about it? What came up for you? What are you going to do with the information you gleaned from the day?

There are many books written about cleansing and fasting and while they all might contain some helpful information, not all of them will be right for you. If, after a while, your inner wisdom isn't guiding you to the right cleansing process for you, then seek the help of a health care professional who is knowledgeable in this area. A good place to start your search for a health care provider in your area is *American Association of Naturopathic Physicians*, 8201 Greensboro Drive/Suite 300, McLean, VA 22102 (phone:703-610-9037; website: www.naturopathic.org). Also, most chiropractic doctors are trained in cleansing procedures.

When you have gathered your list of potential health care providers, make sure you call and interview them first. Find out what experience and training they have. Tell them what you're trying to accomplish and see if they feel comfortable and knowledgeable in this area.

Judy

Judy has endometriosis, a disease where the lining of the uterus grows on the outside of the uterus and other abdominal organs. This can be very painful and cause great difficulty in evacuating the bowel, as well as cause difficulty in digestion and assimilation of nutrients. Judy's case was so severe and debilitating that she'd had surgery to remove the diseased tissue. The doctor reported that there were a lot of adhesions (cord-like structures) holding her small and large intestines very rigidly against the abdominal wall which helped explain her digestive problems and constipation.

She made a choice to start a cleansing program to support her body and then added cleansing herbs, colon hydrotherapy, and body work (in her case, massage) under the supervision of a naturopathic physician. At first, she felt worse instead of better. The toxins were being released into her bloodstream and as a result, she felt tired and ached all over. What surprised her most were all the memories of her childhood that started coming back to her. She came from a very large, poor family and many times during her growing up years; she wasn't nourished physically or emotionally. Junk foods were a treat that eased the pain of this lack of nourishment during her childhood. Now, as an adult with a successful career, she could supply herself with as much comforting junk food as she wanted. But the junk foods along with her disease kept both her body and her psyche in a constant toxic state.

She was committed to doing the work necessary to change these eating patterns and heal her disease. She went to therapy and realized she had a lot of poor self-image issues she had to deal with. She did not love herself or value her life. As Judy worked to cleanse physically and emotionally, she became stronger. Her body slowly began to function better. Her mind was clearer. She was now making choices that honored who she was instead of ones that depleted the value of her life. She now has a much clearer understanding of how her body works and what it's telling her. Today, she is firmly connected to her inner wisdom, and this has brought her a sense of power and freedom she'd never known before.

Support the Eliminative Organs

There are simple things you can do to support the body in its natural cleansing process. Don't allow yourself to become overwhelmed by trying too many new things at one time. For instance, write your intention in your journal to have a healthier body and be in touch with your inner wisdom. Now write down how you are going to do this. For example, take one of the suggestions below and practice it for a month or more until it becomes a natural, everyday thing for you to do. Then add a new, healthy behavior and practice it until that one, too, becomes natural and automatic.

Each time you start something new, write down your intention and what action you're going to do to support that intention. Take time between each new behavior to reflect and record what is happening to you on a physical level as well as what is occurring emotionally. Are you feeling brighter? Are your moods more stabilized? Are old memories working their way to the forefront of your mind? If so, are they pleasant or painful? Does your body crave old habits? Does your body have more energy?

Some of the changes can be very subtle, so if you don't write them down, you might miss them altogether. Kathleen has had clients who, after six months of changes, felt nothing had happened. They hadn't been writing anything down. After she went over their original list of complaints that they'd prepared the first time they'd met with her, they realized a lot of changes *had* occurred. They were quickly becoming so familiar and comfortable with their healthier state of being that they'd completely forgotten how bad they'd felt in the beginning.

Here are some of the things you could do to help cleanse your body:

- Drink ample amounts of pure, filtered water. (Remember, your body needs as a minimum half of its weight in ounces of water every day.)

- Be conscious of the quality and quantity of food you eat. (Eat organic food as much as possible and pay attention not only to portion size, but also to cravings and what is going on emotionally during that time.)

- Take supplements with a good antioxidant to support the ongoing detoxification of the body.

- If you live in a big city or near a chemical plant or a commercial farm, do what you can to address the air quality of your home and workplace.

- Reduce environmental toxins such as cleaning products and reduce your exposure to radiation from such devices microwaves, clocks, computer screens, hair dryers, cell phones, etc.

- Reduce your exposure to parasites by washing all fruits and vegetables before you eat them. (Even organic fruits and vegetables need to be washed thoroughly. Parasites are no dummies. They know a good thing when they crawl up on it!)

- Use toiletries and cosmetics (soaps, shampoos, cosmetics, shaving cream, lotions and moisturizers, etc.) that do not contain harmful chemicals.

Note: If it goes in or on your body, check it out first! In Chapter Seventeen, we provide a resource list of companies that sell clean, environmentally safe products.

17

Finding Clean Food, Water, and Other Healthy Products

Since throughout this book we've talked about a lot of different foods and products, many of which are not commonly found in major grocery stores and department store chains, we wanted to provide you with a resource guide. But remember, just because it's sold in a "health food" store doesn't mean it's necessarily safe. Therefore, don't skip the research part! Besides, doing your own research will undoubtedly lead you to a whole new world of knowledgeable and wonderful people.

This list is not by any means exhaustive, but it is a springboard to get you started making choices for a vital life for yourself and all those with whom you come in contact—including our nurturing Mother Earth.

Organic Foods

The two most common grocery chains in the United States for organic foods are Whole Foods and Wild Oats. Many local grocery chains are starting to have organic food sections, as well. Upon request, your grocer may stock for you the items you desire. It doesn't hurt to ask! Besides, the more they hear such requests, the more likely grocers all over the country will start catering to the demand for healthy, organic, chemical-free foods. Also, see if there are ranches and farms and farmers markets in your area where you can buy healthy food.

- Coleman Natural Beef*, 800-442-8666, 5140 Race Court, Denver, CO 80216, www.colemanbeef.com, for beef products free of added hormones and antibiotics

- Laura's Lean Beef*, 800-487-5326, 2285 Executive Drive/Suite 200, Lexington, KY 40505, www.laurasleanbeef.com, these beef products, too, are free of growth hormones and antibiotics

- Diestel Turkey Ranch*, 209-532-4950, 22200 Lyons Bald Mountain Road, Sonora, CA 95370, www.diestelturkey.com, for turkeys that are organically fed and have never been given antibiotics or hormones

- Petaluma Poultry (Rocky And Rosie Chickens)*, 707-763-1904, 2700 Lakeville Highway, Petaluma, CA 94955, www.petalumapoultry.com, for chickens that have been raised on a 100% vegetarian diet and have not been given any antibiotics and hormones

- Beeler's Pork, 712-533-6042, 235 Oak Street, Brunsville, IA 51008, for clean organic pork

- Horizon Organic Dairy*, 888-494-3020, Boulder CO 80308, www.horizonorganic.com, for a full line of certified organic dairy products

- Organic Valley Farms*, www.organicvalley.com, for organic meat and dairy products

- Diamond Organics, 888-674-2642, www.diamondorganics.com, for organic produce, grains, coffee, teas, and even candy, beer and wine (they will ship food same-day air, freshly picked, and in any quantity)

* *These companies only sell wholesale, but you can contact them for a list of retailers in your area.*

Clean Water in Your Home or Office

First look in your local phone book in the Yellow Pages under "water purifying" and "water filtering" equipment. Do your research and ask for information before being pressured by a sales pitch.

- Harmony, 800-869-3446, www.gaiam.com, for water filters plus a wide variety of products for the home

- Real Goods, 800-762-7325, www.realgoods.com, for a catalog of water filters, plus a variety of other home products

- Natural Lifestyle, 800-752-2775, www.natural-lifestyle.com, for organic food and water filters, earth care products for the home, natural cookware, books and videos

Basic Vitamin & Mineral Supplements

When shopping for vitamin supplements, look for the letters "USP" on the bottle which indicate that the tablets meet the quality and purity standards of the US Pharmacopoeia. Without such an assurance, it's nearly impossible to know the quality of what you are getting, as there are no federal standards regulating the manufacture of supplements.

- Ideal Health, Lynnfield, MA, www.fullbellyonline.com for information. This is one of the best companies we have found for basic vitamin and mineral supplements. You fill out a questionnaire, send in a urine sample, and a personally-tailored, freshly blended formula is sent to you every month.

- Mannatech, Inc., Coppell, TX, for information, www. fullbellyonline.com. This is another company that sells a wide variety of high quality supplements.

Laundry & Household Products

Most health food stores carry environmentally safe laundry and household products, or you can order such products directly from:

- Harmony, 800-869-3446, www.gaiam.com
- Real Goods, 800-762-7325, www.realgoods.com
- Natural Lifestyle, 800-752-2775, www.natural-lifestyle.com

Air Filters for Your Home & Office

Most department stores and hardware stores across the country now carry air filters. If you're unable to find them in your local area, they can be ordered from the following:

- Harmony, 800-869-3446, www.gaiam.com
- Real Goods, 800-762-7325, www.realgoods.com
- Sharper Image, 800-344-4444, www.sharperimage.com

Biological Dentistry

Biological dentistry stresses the use of nontoxic restoration materials for dental work, and focuses on the unrecognized impact dental toxins and hidden dental infections can have on overall health. Here is an organization you may want to contact for information about biological dentistry resources in your area:

- American Academy of Biological Dentistry, P. O. Box 856, Carmel Valley, CA 93924, 831-659-5385 www.biologicaldentistry.org.

Cosmetics, Hair, Skin & Body Care Products

Most health stores sell many safe, natural products. Here are some other resources:

- Real Purity, P.O. Box 307, Grass Lake, MI 49240, 800-253-1694

- Aubrey Organics, Inc., 4419 N. Manhattan Avenue, Tampa, FL 33614, 800-282-7394, www.aubrey-organics.com

Natural Candles

These folks not only make healthy candles, they're are also great on service:

- Way Out Wax Candles, 888-727-1903, www.wayoutwax.com

- Coyote Found Candles, 800-788-4142, www.coyote-found-candles.com

18

An Eight-Day Plan to Get
You Started

When we are beginning something new, it is helpful to have a plan to get started. We have designed an eight-day plan that will help you make a new commitment not just to your body, but to your mind and your spirit as well. True and lasting success will only occur when you address all three.

First, ask yourself, "Why am I doing this? Since it's going to require that I make changes and that I commit time from my already busy life, what will I get from it?"

The answer is more *peace, clarity, balance, an inner sense of freedom, and a feeling that all is well*. How long has it been since you felt that everything was well with you and your body? If you're like so many others, it's been a long, long time. Yet these qualities represent the vitality and health all of us are seeking. Despite our frequent wishes to the contrary, vitality and health don't come in a bottle, by following the latest fad diet, or through a guru.

Vitality and health (and the peace, clarity, balance, inner sense of freedom, and good feelings that accompany them) come from only one place—within. They are your birthright. We were never taught to claim this birthright, however, much less how to reach it. While we might have caught a glimpse of it when we were quite young, what we experienced of our inner wisdom as a child was usually dismissed or disciplined out of us by the age of five. Following this eight-day plan will provide you with the opportunity to rekindle the natural connection that exists between you and your inner wisdom. It will set you moving on the path to recapturing that wonderful "all is well" feeling. Are you ready to start?

The plan begins by writing down what you have been doing. In this way, as you follow the plan and begin making changes, you will become more acutely aware of what your body, thoughts, and feelings are saying to you. As you do the exercises below, you will get to a place where you can decide if your behaviors, thoughts, and beliefs are moving you forward toward your life's goals or if they are keeping them from you and draining you physically and emotionally. This is an exciting journey upon which you are about to embark. Enjoy the whole process as you start making the changes that will work for you.

Your mind, with its incredible warehouse of information, has the power to keep you highly motivated and on track. If mismanaged, however, it can easily and thoroughly sabotage your best intentions. Therefore, it's crucial to your eight-day plan that you start by becoming aware of your habitual thoughts. In order to change them, you need to recognize them and there's no better way than to write them down.

Earlier in this book, we suggested that you record your thoughts and questions, your feelings from the past and present. When you take the time to write (to write to yourself), there is never a right or a wrong way to do it. If you are concerned about your spelling or grammar or have an overriding need to do it correctly, just remember that your journal is for no one to read but you. We think you'll find it more personal, more meaningful if you write by hand rather than doing it on your computer.

When writing in your journal, give yourself permission to list all of the associations that begin to surface from the questions we give you. Resist the temptation to just answer yes or no. Keeping a journal is a way to take all the chatter (especially the negative chatter) out of your mind, put it on paper, and by so doing, to release it. It might be helpful to visualize all those thoughts and words being written instead on a

blackboard that's then wiped clean with an eraser. The surprising benefit of a journal is that you'll find yourself in less conflict with yourself
and the world around you. You'll find you're more able to focus on the
task at hand rather than on your worries and concerns.

We'd also like you to begin writing down your dreams. You may feel
as though you don't dream every night, but in fact you do. It's remembering your dreams that may be new to you. If you are someone who
says you don't remember your dreams, begin by saying instead: "I now
remember my dreams with ease." Place a pad of paper and a pen beside
your bed to record your dreams. (This act alone will help reinforce your
ability to recall your dreams.) Capture them immediately upon waking
before they begin to evaporate. But are dreams all that important?

Dreams, as you might already suspect, can be quite informative.
When you begin this eight-day plan in earnest by sincerely answering
the journal questions, it's likely that old, subconscious feelings will arise
about yourself, your eating habits, and about your body. One of the
most common ways subconscious feelings express themselves is
through dreams. Even though dream images may seem at times totally
unrelated to your reality and even occasionally wild and bizarre, they
often contain within them messages. By honoring your dream state for
the next eight days, you will open up the possibility of remembering
and learning from your dreams. But don't worry about analyzing them.
Allow this journal-keeping exercise to put you in touch with your subconscious mind. You just might open a door to a part of yourself you
didn't know existed.

The spiritual practices we talk about are not about anything religious. They are simply ways to help you communicate more freely with
the spiritual nature that exists within you, within everyone, and within
everything that is alive. You have no doubt seen the pure essence of life
that emanates from eyes that are happy or deeply peaceful. Such eyes
are the windows of spirituality. Spirituality—or life energy, if you prefer—is easy to see in babies, little children, and animals who are well
loved. Our own spiritual nature, which is our connection to life, is most
easily felt when we are quiet in nature or when we take the time to feel

appreciation. Each of the spiritual practices in this eight-day plan encourages you to start by being quiet, going within, and immersing yourself in gratitude.

As you do these exercises, know that you are giving yourself permission to acknowledge your connection to a bigger picture and to experience the deeper context of your life. At some level, that is what we all seek: a feeling of connectedness, of being a meaningful and integral part of the whole of life. When we do this, we feel full—full of life. Unfortunately, we too often attempt to achieve that full feeling of being connected inside through the use/abuse of such inadequate substitutes as food or busy activities. When you follow the spiritual practices we're suggesting, you will experience feelings of fullness that may have been missing from your life when your focus was more primarily on using food in order to feel satisfied.

Anytime we start to make such changes in our life patterns and begin to discover this inner voice, we are automatically making changes to our physical body as well. The food suggestions that follow are here to give you a starting point. As you become more attuned to what your body is saying to you, what you eat will become more individualized and easier to stick to because you will be feeling so much better! You will be balancing your diet so that it supplies your body with all the nutrients it needs to have vitality all the way down to the cellular level. When cells are generating energy and speaking together and efficiently working as one organism, you are operating in a true state of vitality. Temporary bursts of energy should not be confused with the type of vitality we're talking about here.

Everyone needs cellular vitality to be truly healthy and energetic. Cellular vitality gives us the ability to think clearly and the energy to live the life we want. Cellular vitality helps heal injuries and protect us against infections and against such diseases as cancer, arthritis, and diabetes.

The ability to sustain this physical cellular vitality is affected by everything we eat, breathe, drink, and put on our skin, think, and feel. Cells metabolize the nutrients we ingest using oxygen to release the energy they contain. In this process, waste materials are generated which must be removed. Just as it takes energy for our cells to process nutrients, it also takes energy for them to remove waste. So when our energy production (in other words, our very vitality) is compromised within the cells, it starts a downward spiral of declining health.

Only by reclaiming vitality in our cells can we acquire the energy necessary to reverse the process and regain our health. We replenish that vitality by what we do with our lives on a conscious level. Otherwise, we continue to operate completely unaware of what we are doing to our bodies, minds, and spirits. One of the primary objectives of the exercises in this getting-started plan is to help you function more frequently on a conscious level. Journaling is the one of the easiest and best ways to start becoming more aware of what you are doing, thinking, feeling, and eating. But enough talk—let's get started!

The 8-Day Full Heart/Satisfied Belly Spirit—Mind—Body Program
Day One

For Your Spirit—Before you do anything else, go to a quiet room where you won't be distracted by the television, radio, telephones, or family members. Simply sit quietly by yourself for five minutes (set an alarm, if you wish, so you will know when the five minutes are up). Become aware of your breathing. Don't try to change your breathing, just sit comfortably and be cognizant of the feel and gentle sound of your breath. Every once in a while, take a deep breath and let out a relaxed sigh as you exhale. Allow your shoulders and jaw to relax.

For Your Mind—After relaxing, begin writing down what you want to have happen in the next eight days. Don't make it too complicated. Rather, make certain it's something that can be obtained easily in a week (*e.g.,* "I want to feel good about the fact that I made a start"). Write down everything you eat and drink during the day and make some notes about how it makes you feel. (The challenge here will be not to judge it bad or good, but to just record what's happening.) For example, did you get a headache? Did it make you feel moody? Or did it leave you feeling tired and foggy-brained? Pretend you are a fly on the wall watching you. Now that you have an idea of what you've done in the past, let's try something new and see how it makes you feel. Drink eight ounces of filtered water.

For Your Body—To prepare for the next seven days, look at the food plan (below) and make a list of what you will need. When you get home from the grocery store, you can wash and cut up all the fruit and veggies, if you like (it will save you time later). The more efficient you make things for yourself, the more likely you are to follow through with your eight-day plan, especially if you have an already busy schedule. You can also make the soups and cook the meat ahead of time, too.

Day Two

For Your Spirit—Today, find inspiration by reading a passage from any book you enjoy. Read it slowly and, for the next five minutes, contemplate the meaning the message might have in your life. Judge neither the message nor yourself. Just "be with it" and assess how it expresses in your life.

For Your Mind—Drink eight ounces of filtered water while you journal the answers to these questions: How did you sleep last night? Did you have any dreams? (Make a note of them and just observe them and not judge them.) What were your favorite foods as a child? Was the dinner table a safe and comforting place to be? Were you ever criticized for eating too slowly or too fast?

For Your Body—At each meal, take the time to look at the food before you eat it. Pause and observe the colors, the aromas, the textures, how hungry you are, and any other feelings that come up. Write your thoughts in your journal. Again, don't judge yourself. Just write down your-fly-on-the-wall observations. There are no wrong or right answers. Then bless your food and be thankful for it and for the fact that you are on a path to discovering your own inner wisdom. (Here is a sample blessing: "We bless this food and ask that the vibrancy be raised for our highest health. We thank the earth and everyone who has been involved in the creation of this food.")

Breakfast

> 1 8-ounce glass of filtered water
> 2 scrambled eggs with feta cheese and baby spinach
> 1 piece of fruit (*e.g.*, apple, pear, plum, strawberries, melon)—not juice, but rather the whole fruit (and organic, if possible).

Snack

> 1 8-ounce glass of filtered water
> 1 piece of fruit (again, not juice)

Lunch

> 1 8-ounce glass of filtered water
> 2 cups or more of field greens and as many chopped veggies as you want plus 4 ounces of cooked salmon, all topped with your favorite dressing
> Another 8-ounce glass of filtered water after lunch

Snack

> 1 8-ounce glass of filtered water
> 8 to 10 nuts (preferably almonds)—chew each nut one at a time and swallow only when it's completely ground into a paste-like substance
> Another 8-ounce glass of filtered water after snack

Dinner

> 1 8-ounce glass of filtered water
> Steamed vegetable medley topped with a sprinkle of grated cheese
> 1 4-ounce roasted chicken breast
> Cucumber, dill, and yogurt salad

Note: if you are used to drinking beverages containing caffeine (*e.g.*, coffee, sodas, etc.), you may continue to do so, but drink them in addition to the water we're suggesting.

Throughout the day, write down how you felt when you ate, what your mood was, whether you felt satisfied, and whether you went to the bathroom more than usual. Record in your journal if you liked what you ate or did this whole process annoyed you. Did you wish instead there were a magic pill you could take?

Day Three

For Your Spirit—Think of someone who has touched your life in a meaningful way and spend five minutes by yourself in reflection on his or her contribution to the person you are today.

For Your Mind—Drink eight ounces of filtered water while you journal the answers to these questions: How did you sleep last night? Did you dream? (Again, just make a note about your dreams and don't attempt to figure them out.) Up until now, who has been your authority on what you ate and when? Who has been your authority on how your body looks?

For Your Body—Go for a ten-minute walk or follow your exercise program. Observe what you see, smell, and feel. What did you think about when you were alone? At each meal, take the time to look at the food before eating it. Pause and observe the colors, the smells, the textures, how hungry you are, and any other feelings or thoughts that come up for you. Write these observations in your journal and do so without judging them. Remember, there are no wrong or right answers. Then bless your food and be thankful for it and for the fact that you are on a path to discovering your own inner wisdom.

Breakfast

> 1 8-ounce glass of filtered water
> 1/2-cup cottage cheese topped with fresh or frozen organic berries
> Celery and carrot sticks with almond or peanut butter

Snack

> 1 8-ounce glass of filtered water
> 1 piece of fruit

Lunch

> 1 8-ounce glass of filtered water
> Steamed green beans
> Small baked yam or sweet potato
> 4 ounces of shrimp sautéed in olive oil and garlic
> Another 8-ounce glass of filtered water after lunch

Snack

> 1 8-ounce glass of filtered water
> Tomato sliced in half with a small piece of mozzarella or goat cheese on each half
> Another 8-ounce glass of filtered water after snack

Dinner

> 1 8-ounce glass of filtered water
> Green lettuce salad (at least 2 cups) and as many chopped veggies as you want, plus an avocado, a couple of chopped nuts, and balsamic vinegar and olive oil dressing

Write down throughout the day how you felt when you ate. Continue to note what your mood was, what your energy level was, whether you felt satisfied, and indicate whether you ate any food that wasn't on the plan. If you ate something not on the plan, what conversation did you have with yourself when you did that? Just observe. Don't judge. Whatever it was, it was neither bad nor good. Rather, it's just a behavior with belief systems wrapped around it. It can be changed if it no longer serves you. This program is a process and not a one-time fix. The important thing here is simply to become aware so that you start to see what behaviors and beliefs are running your life.

If you didn't exercise in the morning, do so before dinner. Observe what you smell, hear, see, and feel as you exercise. Movement changes your body. Your body was made to move and the chemicals in your brain that make you feel good are activated with movement.

Day Four

For Your Spirit—Today, find something in your house or outside environment that is pleasing to you and contemplate its attractiveness for five minutes. Simply appreciate it and spend some time being with that one object. If you find your mind drifting off to other thoughts or objects, gently bring your attention back to the one thing you have chosen for today.

For Your Mind—Drink eight ounces of filtered water while you journal the answers to these questions: How did you sleep last night? How are your feelings and your desire for food connected? Do you sometimes want to eat when you're upset? Are there perhaps other times when you're upset that you can't stand the thought of food? In the past, what feelings and behaviors have been connected to difficult situations for you?

For Your Body—At each meal, remember to take the time to look at the food before you eat it. Pause and observe the colors, the smells, the textures, how hungry you are, and any other feelings or thoughts you might have, and write down what you observe. Remind yourself once again not to judge your thoughts. Just write down your fly-on-the-wall observations. Then bless your food and be thankful for it and the fact you are on a path to discovering your own inner wisdom and guidance.

Breakfast

    1 8-ounce glass of filtered water
    Scrambled tofu (or eggs) with mixed chopped veggies, salsa, and olives
    1 piece of fruit

Snack

    1 8-ounce glass of filtered water
    1 piece of fruit

Lunch

> 1 8-ounce glass of filtered water
> 2 cups or more of green lettuce or spinach, with as many chopped veggies as you want, plus 4 ounces of roasted turkey breast with seeds and dressing
> Another 8-ounce glass of filtered water after lunch

Snack

> 1 8-ounce glass of filtered water
> Green pepper and celery strips with some almond or peanut butter
> Another 8-ounce glass of filtered water after snack

Dinner

> 1 8-ounce glass of filtered water
> Sautéed green and yellow squash with tomato, onion, and garlic
> Steamed asparagus (or other green veggie)

Broiled 4-ounce lean steak (or if you don't want red meat, substitute chicken patty burger)

Day Five

For Your Spirit—Spend at least ten minutes today listening to music or to the sounds of nature. Don't do anything else but listen. Don't criticize yourself if your mind wanders. Instead, just notice that you have mentally wandered away and gently bring yourself back to the sounds around you. Afterwards, make a few notes to yourself about how you felt.

For Your Mind—Drink eight ounces of filtered water while you journal the answers to these questions: How did you sleep last night? (Write down any dreams without judgment or trying to figure them out.) How often do you crave food? What foods have you craved? Looking back without judgment, were you hungry when you craved the food? Did you let yourself get too hungry? As you contemplate the answers to these questions, do you see any patterns of when you crave certain foods?

For Your Body—Go for a ten-minute or longer walk or follow your exercise program. Observe. What thoughts arose as you were moving? At each meal, take time to look closely at your food before eating it. Write in your journal about these observations and your thoughts. Bless your food and be thankful for the journey upon which you've embarked that will help you connect to the guidance that makes *you* the authority in your life.

Breakfast

1 8-ounce glass of filtered water
Smoothie (put in blender: 1/2-cup of cottage cheese or 1 cup of plain yogurt, and add strawberries, raspberries, or blueberries or all three—add some filtered water if too thick or a couple of ice cubes and blend)

Snack

1 8-ounce glass of filtered water
1 piece of fruit

Lunch

1 8-ounce glass of filtered water
4 ounces of broiled white flaky-type fish
Steamed artichoke
Sautéed carrots and snow peas
Another 8-ounce glass of filtered water after lunch

Snack

1 8-ounce glass of filtered water
Salsa and cut-up veggies
Another 8-ounce glass of filtered water after snack

Dinner

> 1 8-ounce glass of filtered water
> Tabbouleh and hummus with 1 whole-wheat pita
> 2 cups or more of mixed greens plus chopped veggies, seeds, feta cheese, olives, and dressing

Continue to write down how you feel. What thoughts are you having about your food, your body, your career, your friends, your family, and your peers? Are you feeling satisfied? Did you feel energetic or sluggish today?

Day Six

For Your Spirit—Today, do a walking meditation. Set aside time to walk for at least ten to fifteen minutes, preferably outside in a beautiful place. Rather than thinking about other things, allow your thoughts to be entirely with you on this walk. Be aware of your feet as they touch the ground. Feel the temperature of the air on your skin. Notice the sounds around you. Keep yourself in the present moment. When you're done, spend a few minutes writing in your journal about how that experience felt.

For Your Mind—Drink eight ounces of filtered water while you journal the answers to these questions: How did you sleep last night? Did you have any dreams? (Observe your dreams without judging them.) What is the most common thought you have about what has to happen in order for you to be happy? (e.g., I'll be happy when I have more time or when I have more money or when I lose ten pounds, etc.)

For Your Body—Exercise or go for a ten-minute or more walk. Be observant of your body and your thoughts, as well as your surroundings. What thoughts came up for you as you moved your body? At each meal, take note of your mood and of your food before eating it. Bless your food and be thankful for it and for your progress toward being in touch with your inner wisdom.

Breakfast

> 1 8-ounce glass of filtered water
> Broccoli omelet
> 1 piece of fruit

Snack

> 1 8-ounce glass of filtered water
> 1 piece of fruit

Lunch

> 1 8-ounce glass of filtered water
> Chicken and veggie soup
> Caesar salad
> Another 8-ounce glass of filtered water after lunch

Snack

> 1 8-ounce glass of filtered water
> 2 king crab legs with lemon
> Another 8-ounce glass of filtered water after snack

Dinner

> 1 8-ounce glass of filtered water
> 4 ounces of lean red meat or turkey patty
> Steamed cabbage and butter
> Small baked yam or sweet potato

Write down throughout the day how you felt when you ate and how you felt about an hour after eating. How were your moods? Your energy levels? Did you feel satisfied? Did you eat food that wasn't on the food plan? What mental "conversations" did you have with and about yourself? Again, write down what comes to you. Just be an observer and not a judge.

Day Seven

For Your Spirit—Close your eyes and practice relaxing for ten minutes. Do this sitting up in a comfortable position. Set your timer so you don't have to worry about the time. With your eyes closed, imagine that you are a pat of butter in the sun and all the tension throughout your body is simply melting away. Drop your conscious awareness from behind your eyes down through your body to the balance point (about 2 inches below your belly button). If you can't move it that far down, bring it as far down from your head as possible. Focus on the gentle rise and fall of your belly as you breathe. Continue to let the tension melt away. When your ten minutes are up, make a few notes as to how that exercise felt. (When you get good at this, you can get the equivalent of an hour of sleep simply by relaxing deeply for ten minutes!)

For Your Mind—Drink eight ounces of filtered water while you write out the answer to this question: What would you eat and drink if *you* really mattered? Throughout the rest of the day, periodically ask yourself that question.

For Your Body—Remember to observe the details of your food at each meal before eating. Pause and observe the colors, the aromas, the textures, how hungry you are, and any other feelings or thoughts that arise. Write down what you observe. Again, there are no wrong or right answers. Then bless your food and be thankful for it and the fact you are on a path to discovering your connection to yourself.

Breakfast

> 1 8-ounce glass of filtered water
> 3 Wasa sesame rye crackers with goat cheese and smoked salmon
> 1 piece of fruit

Snack

> 1 8-ounce glass of filtered water
> Cut-up veggies and dressing dip

Lunch

> 1 8-ounce glass of filtered water
> 4 ounces of tuna on a bed of greens (2 cups or more) and as many chopped veggies as you want, plus dressing
> Another 8-ounce glass of filtered water after lunch

Snack

> 1 8-ounce glass of filtered water
> 1 piece of fruit
> Another 8-ounce glass of filtered water after snack

Dinner

> 1 8-ounce glass of filtered water
> Lamb or turkey and veggie stew
> Spinach salad with turkey bacon and dressing

Write down throughout the day how you felt when you ate. Note your various moods and corresponding energy levels. Were you satisfied with your meals or did you find yourself craving certain foods? If so, what was going on in your life at the times of these cravings? What type of chatter is going on in your head about what you are doing? Just observe and write down what you are seeing.

Day Eight

For Your Spirit—Congratulations! You have followed the "Full Heart/Satisfied Belly Spirit—Mind—Body Program" for seven days. The more you do it, the easier it gets. In recognition of your accomplishments of the past week, today list at least 25 things, people, feelings, or anything else for which you feel grateful. Don't think about them too much. Just write them down. In the future, whenever you are feeling discouraged about something, doing this exercise can help you shift your perspective.

For Your Mind—Drink eight ounces of filtered water while you write the following affirmations at least 21 times: "I now accept my need for love and connection that food will never fill. And I now lovingly accept that everything I put in my mouth affects me emotionally, physically, and spiritually." Next, write down how you slept last night and any dreams you had. And, no, you're not to judge them! Just observe them.

For Your Body—Go for at least a ten-minute walk or follow your exercise program. Observe what you see, hear, smell, and feel. What thoughts arose as you were moving your body? At each meal, take the time to look at the food before eating it. Pause and observe everything about it. Make note of how hungry you are and of any feelings and thoughts you might be having. Don't judge—just write! Then bless your food and be thankful for it and the fact that you are on a fascinating path of self-discovery.

Breakfast

  1 8-ounce glass of filtered water
  1 bowl of oatmeal and a poached egg
  1 piece of fruit

Snack

  1 8-ounce glass of filtered water
  Veggie sticks and almond or peanut butter

Lunch

  1 8-ounce glass of filtered water
  2 corn taco shells filled with ground chicken or turkey, taco seasoning, tomatoes, green peppers, and onions
  Garden salad
  Another 8-ounce glass of filtered water after lunch

Snack

> 1 8-ounce glass of filtered water
> 1 piece of fruit
> Another 8-ounce glass of filtered water after snack

Dinner

> 1 8-ounce glass of filtered water
> Stir fry with 4 ounces of fish and veggies
> Garden salad
> Small piece of dessert (your choice!)

Write down what came up for you during the day. How were your moods and energy levels? Were you satisfied? What thoughts and self-talk went on during the day? Can you remember what you ate? Don't judge your observations; just write them down. Remember there is no right or wrong. The goal is to discover your inner wisdom, for that is the authority that governs who you are and how you are to eat.

Feel good about yourself, for you have finished eight days of discovery!

Now, go back and read your journal for clues from your body and your inner self that will help you better understand what worked for you and what didn't. Ask yourself a few more questions:

1. By the end of the week, were you finding yourself thirsty when it was time to drink water again? (When the body is dehydrated, the thirst mechanism often gets turned off.)

2. Did you want the snacks? None of them or maybe only one? Did you find that the fruit gave you more energy in the morning or the afternoon?

3. Did certain foods affect your mood and energy level?

4. Was it hard for you to be alone with yourself for five or ten minutes each day? What do you typically do to fill up that space of time?

5. Did certain foods make you feel more mentally clear?

6. How did it feel to move your body? Did your body start wanting more movement?

7. Did you crave foods on certain days? What foods did you crave? What was going on in your life at the time?

8. Throughout these practices, when did you feel the most connected to yourself and your surroundings?

9. Did you have any headaches or other aches and pains during the last eight days? Did previous aches and pains go away? Were these associated with food or circumstances in your day?

10. Looking back through your journal entries, what has been your greatest insight?

Now write down what you want to do next week based on what you've learned about yourself. Keep observing and adjusting what and how much you're eating by how satisfied, energetic, and stable your moods and energy levels are. With time, you will be doing this automatically with each meal. Your inner wisdom and body language will speak to you about what works for you and what doesn't. You will have become your own guru. What a gift you will have given yourself—a *Full Heart/Satisfied Belly*.

III

Introduction

Now that you are using the suggestions outlined in Part II, you are more aware of your thoughts and feelings. You are becoming more confident in your choices of food and how you view yourself. Your thoughts and beliefs about your body are changing. You are acquiring better insights and the ability to act accordingly because of them. Congratulations! That's wonderful!

Things are going along smoothly and then you go on a fantastic cruise, or your boss isn't happy with your work, or your schedule is overloaded, or you have a crisis in the family. As a result, you find yourself slipping back into old destructive patterns and when that happens, familiar guilt and punishment once again rear their ugly heads. What are you to do?

The chapters in this last section will help you reinforce your ability to reconnect to your inner wisdom during these inevitable challenging times. You will learn that what you have done in the past does not have to repeat and become your current experience, *unless you choose it to be*. You will learn how to recognize the feelings that arise during difficult times, how to effectively deal with those feelings, and how to release them. You will be reminded to trust yourself and your faithful inner guidance system (to which you are always connected), even when you feel as though you've made a mistake. The path of trusting yourself and your process brings you a deeper connection with yourself, and thus a deeper fulfillment.

During these times, listen and you may hear yourself judging your behavior as "bad" or "good," depending on what you have eaten. Often that negative chatter is an unconscious habit. You may automatically be feeling wrong, guilty, or ashamed—all based simply on what you ate that day.

That habit of allowing your self-esteem to waver based on what you put in your mouth is destructive and traps you by continually pulling you back into old habits. The chapters in this last section will teach you how to catch yourself in the act of thinking what we call "backsliding" thoughts so that you can realign your thoughts and feelings. Being in charge of your thought processes gives you the internal power to make better choices so you can thoroughly enjoy eating free of guilt.

In order to maintain your new positive life behavior, you must first learn to deal with the hidden thoughts, feelings, and energy that were responsible for creating your past behavior in the first place. In Part III, we will lead you through exercises and examples that will help you learn to release buried feelings so you can stay on track with the positive changes you're making in your life. A big part of these positive changes is rearranging your life so that there is less focus on what you eat. You will find that when food no longer controls your life, you have more space and more energy to devote to new activities, exercise, fun, and relating with others.

Learning how to approach emotionally challenging situations without using food as a drug is one of the first steps toward lasting freedom. When you can see all these situations as teachers instead of as threats, you are then in the position of a student who is ready and willing to learn and change. When you achieve that level of understanding, you no longer have to feel embarrassed about yourself if occasionally you don't do it perfectly. Instead of causing those old bugaboos of confusion and guilt, challenges can be seen as the learning experiences that they are.

In this section, you will learn new ways to relate to any circumstance, whether it is a pleasure cruise where you are daily confronted with buffets loaded with fat and refined carbohydrates, a family reunion where the picnic table is piled high with all your favorite childhood foods, or the trauma of losing someone close to you. You will be shown ways in which you can relate to the raw experiences of life without using food as an anesthetic. We challenge you to shift your experience from living in old patterns of repeated failures to seeing life as a gift and as a journey of joyful experiences.

Part III covers:

- Backsliding as a learning experience

- Developing activities that are not based on food

- Learning how to maintain your new self-image

- Learning how to eat well in circumstances other than your normal daily routine

- Allowing yourself to eat the foods you love without guilt and shame

19

Beating Backsliding

We've known very few people in our practices that have started healthy new habits of living and eating without experiencing at least some backsliding in which they fell back into old patterns of behavior. People frequently get motivated and make positive changes in their lives. Then, for any number of reasons, they have a brief relapse, and that first relapse leads to a second relapse and before they have really made a conscious decision to do so, they are solidly entrenched once again in their old behaviors.

When this happens, their reaction is to say, "See? I knew it. I just can't do this. It's too hard." And then they give up making any changes, at least for a while. After a few months or years, they may try again and then end up repeating the whole process. Many people spend their entire lives in this endless cycle of attempting to change their behavior but still feeling dissatisfied, which causes them to fail once again.

The best way to approach backsliding is to expect it. Once you learn to expect it, you can plan for it. What happens when you do this is that when you make a conscious choice to eat something that is not your normal fare, you can go back to your healthier way of eating without punishing yourself or feeling guilty.

Studies have shown that which we all knew or suspected already: healthy eaters sometimes eat poorly and occasionally overeat. The difference is that truly healthy eaters don't beat themselves up afterwards. Neither do they deprive themselves of certain foods by declaring, for example, that they will never eat another cookie or donut again as long as they live. Healthy eaters are aware that the moment they begin to have critical, negative thoughts about themselves, the destructive cycle has begun. Remember, you are more apt to backslide when you're being hard on yourself than when you're feeling good about yourself.

So how do you plan for backsliding instead of just waiting for it to happen? You begin by moving the act of backsliding out of the realm of denial and gradually become more aware of your behavior. Once you do that, you will have a host of choices before you. One of Linda's clients serves as a good example.

Ralph

Ralph went to the grocery store to buy diapers for his baby. As soon as he got there, however, he had an intense craving for chocolate chip ice cream. That was not all that unusual, as chocolate chip ice cream had always been one of his favorite foods. In an attempt to improve his eating habits, however, he had chosen to completely eliminate ice cream from his daily diet. As Ralph walked through the store that day, he suddenly became obsessed with thoughts about ice cream. He jokingly said that he could almost hear it seductively calling his name.

Ralph told Linda that he used to eat a quart of ice cream in one sitting. Therefore, he had anticipated that ice cream would prove to be an enormous temptation because it had been such a big part of his life. Before he got married, he used to say that ice cream was his best friend. Now that he was happily married and had a new baby, he no longer wanted his relationship with ice cream to have that much importance in his life.

He'd gone three months since he last tasted that cold, sweet substance, and his memories and feelings about it remained painfully vivid that day as he walked through the grocery store. He knew how he handled this craving would be very important. He mentally reviewed what Linda had told him about backsliding. He stopped there, right in the middle of the aisle, and thought about it. After a moment or two, he made a conscious decision to let himself have a little of his favorite ice cream. He bought the smallest portion available, took it home, ate it slowly and mindfully, and allowed himself to enjoy it completely without any reservations or guilt. He said later that he had never before enjoyed ice cream as much as he did that evening!

The best part was that he was completely satisfied without one speck of guilt, and continued on his food plan the next day. Knowing that he could occasionally have his favorite treat relaxed his fears of eating well on a daily basis. Ralph made an agreement with himself that he would not backslide for any food that wasn't as good and satisfying as his favorite ice cream. If someone offered him a sweet food at a party that he wasn't particularly crazy about, he could make a conscious choice to say "no, thank you." He reserved the right to give himself permission for special treats for things he really liked. Ralph had planned for his backsliding, even if it was just before it happened. He took a few minutes to think about what was really going on before he acted.

Another way to plan ahead is to decide in advance when you are going to have a favorite treat. In addition, you must also plan ahead about how you will handle the most common feelings that can precipitate backsliding. Many times, especially when we are in denial, we don't really think about what we want to eat. When we move into awareness, we can begin the process of checking in with what we want in the present moment. Birthday cake is a good example.

Linda says that birthday cake is not one of her favorite foods, despite the fact that for years she accepted and ate cake on her birthdays. Later, as she became more acutely aware of her relationship with food, Linda began letting her family and friends know that cake was not something she really wanted to eat on her birthday. She soon came to realize that she rarely wanted dessert of any kind. Today, she will occasionally order a special dessert after a meal and share it with the people she's eating with. She says that approach gives her a taste of something special she enjoys without overindulging. As she learned to listen to her body, she discovered that one bite too many of any good meal can often spoil the whole experience.

In addition to being critical of yourself, there are other feelings that can create a mentality ripe for backsliding. Rebellion is one of the emotions that must be taken into consideration. After you have successfully mastered eating in a more healthy way and are regularly checking in with your body to hear what it needs, you may begin to have rebellious thoughts.

Remember Linda's client Rochelle who ate birthday cake at her niece's party? Rebellion played a role in that impulsive decision. People often don't recognize rebellion for what it is. Instead, they conjure up countless rationalizations for why they deviated from a carefully designed food plan. Once the rationalizations are swept away, it is often discovered that the primary cause is rebellion. There is a way, however, to get ahead of those rebellious feelings and remain in control.

For one thing, you already know what your favorite food treats are. Allowing yourself to integrate them in smaller portions (as Ralph did when he had a small amount of ice cream rather than an entire quart) will often be enough to remind you that you truly are not being deprived and therefore don't need to rebel. If you love chocolate, for example, here is something you can do. Buy one piece of the finest chocolate you can find (most shopping malls have chocolatiers that offer exceptionally good chocolate). Sit down and enjoy it. Allow yourself to be totally satisfied. When you take your time and fully experience the pleasure and taste, there is no need to rebel.

Boredom of eating the same thing over and over again can also cause backsliding. It's very easy to fall into a habit of eating the same healthy food on a daily basis. That's why it is important to try new and unique foods and food combinations. If you don't, you are almost assured of suffering from "eating boredom." What is a natural desire for a variety in your diet can then initiate a backsliding event. Your palate thrives on a host of different tastes. A monotonous, unchanging diet is a certain recipe for boredom.

Boredom is often another aspect of denial or an unwillingness to take a risk. If you are feeling bored, it may have very little to do with what you are eating. Be honest with yourself now, for there is probably a bigger issue afoot. Is there something you have to say to someone and you're dreading the confrontation? Is there some risk you need to take that you are avoiding? What project are you procrastinating? Rigorously examine everything about yourself and your life, and see whether or not boredom is affecting your food choices. Too often, we act out in rebellion to avoid boredom. We do it in small ways, such as eating, rather than looking at what is really going on with us in our lives.

Whenever it occurs, just remember that backsliding is a clue that you can use to help you decipher what's going on with you emotionally. No matter how tempting the food might be, when you are in complete integration with yourself, feeling balance in your life, and dedicated to your highest and best health, it is easy to say no to that which doesn't work for you, whether that is food or any other choice that comes along. That's why being able to determine what is really going on for you emotionally and physically is an essential component in your ability to feel your *Full Heart/Satisfied Belly*.

Linda says that when she was grieving her parents' deaths, it took her some time before she regained her emotional balance. When she did, however, her diet and exercise program returned to normal. Similarly, as Ralph became more accustomed to living his life without large doses of refined sugar, he craved it less and less. He was in better balance physically and emotionally and therefore able to handle his backsliding without either punishing himself or going "off the wagon."

So anytime you backslide, you need to ask yourself what is really going on with you. Here are some questions to ask yourself and some suggestions to start the process of solving each situation:

- Have I been getting enough sleep lately? How do I need to improve my sleeping patterns? Maybe I need to go to bed earlier or not eat before bedtime or calm my mind that is either spinning or worrying too much. Do I need to get a professional medical opinion?

- Do I feel pressured about something in my life? If so, what? Am I procrastinating? Am I afraid or do I really need more time? What assertive steps do I need to take to resolve the pressure?

- Do I feel criticized by someone or by myself? Is there a seed of truth in the criticism I'm receiving? What is my responsibility in the matter? Am I being too hard on myself? How can I be gentler with myself?

- Am I taking my vitamins or prescription drugs on a regular basis? If not, why not? Create a ritual or a habit to make sure you take care of yourself properly and lovingly.

- Am I feeling lonely? Is there a relationship problem in my life that needs to be confronted? Do I need to take a risk in order to make friends, tell the truth, or create a social connection? What's keeping me from doing that right now?

- Am I working too hard? If so, why am I doing that? Am I willing to change my lifestyle to make time for myself? Is there some way I can take more breaks or more frequent days off?

- Am I feeling angry or resentful? What is it that I need to let go of or confront?

- Am I sad about an event or disappointed in something or someone else? Have I made myself clear about what I expected or wanted? Do I have a habit of expecting too much from myself or others? Do I need to cry? Do I need to be more assertive about what I want and need?

These questions will go a long way toward helping you achieve a deeper knowledge of yourself and your motives, especially when you backslide without planning for it. There is always more going on emotionally than you might be aware of. Backsliding, when seen as a symptom or a clue, can lead you to a richer, more meaningful understanding of yourself. If you are willing to see backsliding as a gift rather than a punishment, you can use it to help you guide your life as you maintain your new self-image.

20

Maintaining Your New Self-Image

Improving the way you look on the outside is a wonderful experience. Every time you see yourself in the mirror, you'll be reminded of how well you are doing. If you've lost a few pounds, you'll be able to wear new clothes. If you have finally managed to gain some sorely needed weight, you will be able to see your health returning. With all that positive verification and excitement, it's quite natural to assume that you'll be able maintain that wonderful, new image without any difficulty. There are, however, challenges that must be dealt with in order to sustain your success, because it takes time to heal the emotional reasons that led to your situation in the first place. If old patterns are not permanently changed, your previous behavior will almost assuredly return with a vengeance at some point.

Sarah and Charlie

This couple illustrates the importance of attending to the deeper feelings beneath a new physical change. A forty-year-old mother of two, Sarah lost sixty pounds in ten weeks by using a liquid diet drink. Having been overweight as both a young child and a teenager, she had never looked as good as she did at forty. Her friends barely recognized her! She was so excited with her new body that she went on a shopping spree and bought sexy clothes she'd never dared wear before. Her husband, Charlie, was also excited about her weight loss, and understandably so, for their previously lackluster sex life had greatly improved.

Having always been shy because of her weight, a new and extroverted Sarah emerged. For the first time in her life, she found herself the center of male attention and discovered a host of feelings she had never before experienced. She was enjoying her new-found allure. At the same time, however, she felt terribly self-conscious. As for Charlie, he was even more uncomfortable than was Sarah with all the new attention she was getting. They began to argue about everything but the real, underlying issue. As the arguments continued and the irritability between them grew, Sarah found herself gradually becoming attracted to another man. She was so startled by having sexual feelings for someone other than her husband that she broke all the rules of her maintenance diet and binged on junk food for five days in a row!

At her next checkup, Sarah found she'd gained six pounds. Even though the doctor warned her about returning to her old eating habits, Sarah couldn't seem to control her craving for junk food. Though she felt guilty about it, she continued to eat compulsively. As she gained more and more weight, men began to find her less attractive. She had succeeded in burying her feelings in fries and hamburgers. Charlie began to relax as he got his shy, introverted, overweight wife back. You see, Charlie's insecurity was also buried in Sarah's extra pounds. By the time Sarah gained all her weight back (plus ten pounds more), their marriage was just as it had been before—dead but safe.

Sarah and Charlie are perfect examples of what can happen when the deeper issues surrounding the initial weight gain are not dealt with effectively. Both of them were very insecure. Sarah longed for more emotional intimacy and craved physical connection with Charlie, but was repeatedly rejected by him. Sarah, a middle child in a large family, had always felt overlooked and that she'd never received the attention she wanted from her parents.

Charlie was not an affectionate person by nature, and seldom touched Sarah in any loving or sensual way. Charlie, too, had felt insecure all his life. His parents were intelligent and logical, but not at all demonstrative with their affection. They never kissed him goodnight or gave him hugs or compliments. They were, however, very vocal and free with their criticism. It is no surprise then that Charlie was insecure in his ability to be a good lover. Rather than face the issue directly, he withdrew his affections from Sarah. As a matter of fact, he had always thought it a miracle that Sarah had fallen in love with him in the first place and had agreed to marry him. He saw himself as unattractive and therefore undesirable. When his wife began to regain the weight she'd lost, he felt more comfortable and less threatened, because he assumed she would be less attractive to other men.

Sarah first came to see Linda because she was depressed. As her therapy developed, it became clear that there were important relationship issues that needed to be addressed. To Sarah's relief, Charlie agreed to begin couple's therapy. It wasn't easy for either one of them. But as the real issues began to emerge, it became clear that each was starved for the other's attention. At first, they learned to recognize their own feelings, and then they learned how to communicate those emotions to one other. They were surprised to learn that the other was also feeling insecure.

Eventually, Sarah was able to express her anger toward Charlie for rejecting her sexually. Charlie began to deal with his own issues of feelings of sexual inferiority and gradually began reaching out to Sarah for physical touch and intimacy. While their marital state was healing, Sarah began a basic food plan. In contrast to her first time, she now began to lose weight gradually. A year after they began therapy, they both felt much happier in the marriage and Sarah had not only lost pounds, but also the insecurity that the extra weight was hiding. Charlie was able to support her this time, because he felt better about himself and about their marriage.

The only reason they were able to get to the bottom of their marital problems was that they were both willing to look more deeply. It takes courage to look within at feelings you've ignored most of your life. It's very important to remember that any addiction (alcohol, drugs, food, etc.) is just a symptom, and never the whole story.

Looking back at your history of weight gain and loss, health challenges, and injuries is a way to uncover emotional patterns. You probably have a personal pattern of behavior that has been consistent, even if you've never looked at it before. In order to maintain your new image, it is important to be aware of your history so you can more quickly and effectively address the hidden feelings that may otherwise sabotage your new sense of yourself.

On page 225, you will find a graph titled *Your Health & Accident History*. To use this graph, first list on a separate sheet of paper all your significant health challenges, injuries, and weight fluctuations, and how old you were at the time each of these occurred. Next, rate each entry on a scale of one to ten as to how traumatic each experience was for you (1 = the least traumatic, 10 = the most traumatic). Rate each experience relative to the others you have listed.

Tommy

Here's how one of Linda's clients gathered this information about his own life (note the ratings he assigned):

AGE	EVENT	RATING
4 years old	Tricycle accident	2
6 years old	Bicycle accident	3
8 years old	Rock climbing incident—head injury	6
12 years old	Badly twisted ankle at summer camp	6
15 years old	Skiing accident—broken wrist	4
18 years old	Motorcycle accident	9
19 years old	Gained twenty-five pounds	5
22 years old	Lost twenty-pounds	0
24 years old	Gained thirty pounds	8

When Tommy was a little boy of four, he fell off his tricycle and into a ditch. It was the most traumatic event of his young life and if at the time you'd asked him how upset he was, he would have said it was definitely a ten. Years later, Tommy had a motorcycle accident and was in the hospital for two weeks. His left leg was badly damaged and despite undergoing physical therapy for several months, he continued to walk with a slight limp. Because he was still affected by the motorcycle accident when he filled out his health and injury graph, he rated the tricycle accident as a two on the scale of his overall life trauma and the motorcycle accident a nine. He told Linda that he rated the weight gain an eight because he felt so uncomfortable, got teased by his coworkers, and was convinced that the extra pounds made it impossible for him to attract the best-looking girls.

Once you've written down your own health history list and your ratings, it's time to put them on the graph. The age you were at the time of the experience is at the bottom, starting with birth (on the left) and increasing horizontally in five-year increments to your current age (on the right). On the left vertical side of the graph, you will see "one" at the bottom and "ten" at the top. That scale is the level of upset you perceive you experienced from that event.

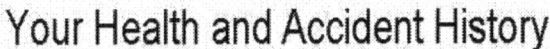

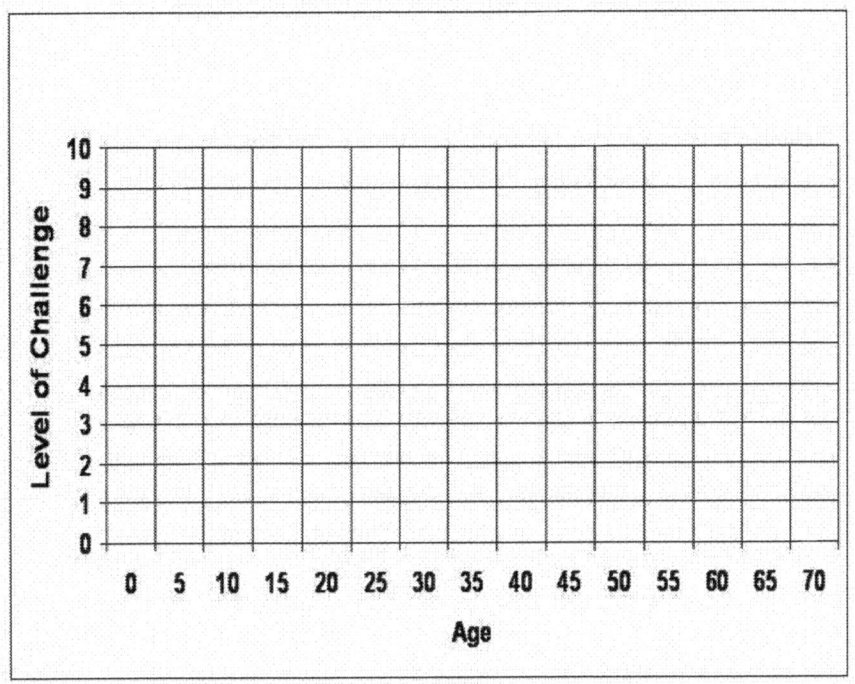

Next, place a dot on the graph at the intersection of your age and level of upset about your first illness, accident, or weight change. Then move on to the next incident. Continue to place dots on your graph as you move through your list of life experiences. When you're done, connect the dots and create your graph. Now look at your graph and try to remember what was going on in your life emotionally at the time of each of the life events you've listed. Write down as much as you can recall about the emotional climate you were experiencing when these events happened.

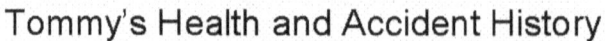

Tommy's Health and Accident History

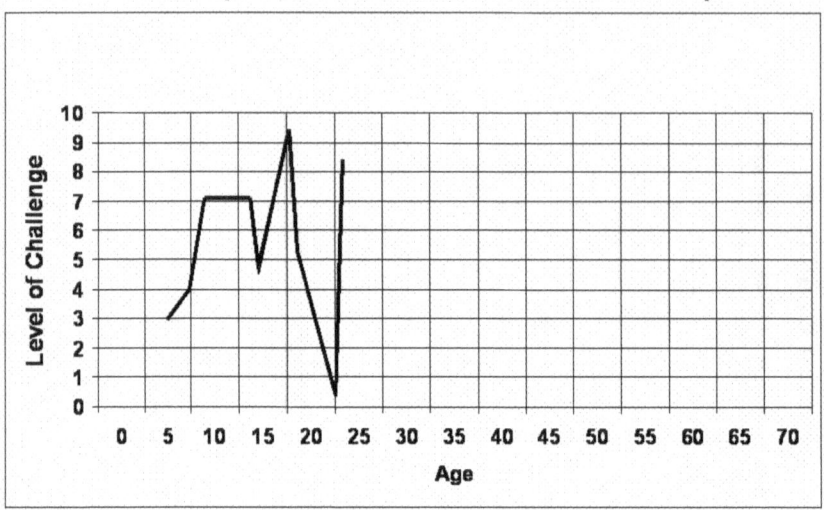

When Tommy finished his graph, he noticed a pattern of highs and lows had occurred every two years or so. When he went back and added the emotional information behind the events on his graph, he discovered that each time he'd had a serious accident or gained weight, he had felt abandoned and/or rejected in some way.

Linda was curious to know what had been going on in his household when he had the tricycle accident at four years old. She had a hunch that the pattern that seemed to govern his life might have begun at that time. Tommy, however, had only a few faint memories of his life before the age of ten. Linda suggested they go back through imagery and visualization to see if they could uncover what else was happening on that day he fell in the ditch. With curiosity, he decided to give it a try.

With Linda's help, this grown man who said he had no conscious memories of the early years of his life was able to go right back to the day of his first accident. As he watched the events unfold, he realized that was the first time in his life his mother had left him to go to work. He sat in Linda's office and "watched" that little boy sobbing as his mother left and he experienced again how depressed and abandoned he had felt. In an attempt to cheer him up that afternoon, his baby-sitter had suggested he go outside and ride his tricycle. Although he was crying and only wanted to stay inside and play, he did as she said and went out and got on his tricycle. Blinded by his tears, he didn't watch where he was going and he careened off the edge of the sidewalk right into a ditch. Fortunately, the baby-sitter saw him fall and was able to rescue him right away. Nonetheless, Tommy was thoroughly traumatized. He longed to be held and comforted, preferably by his mother. He might have even accepted affection from the baby-sitter, but he barely knew her and she didn't appear to be a warm and fuzzy type of person. He also didn't want her to know that he was feeling like a baby. So he pretended he was okay.

So what does this have to do with his health and accident pattern? Tommy's pain at having his mother leave him all day for the first time got connected to the trauma of his tricycle accident. In reality, they were two entirely separate incidents; but because they happened one right after one another, they got unconsciously linked together. As he looked back at his history on the graph, he saw that every time he felt major rejection or abandonment, he suffered an injury or some other type of setback. Two separate experiences of life—emotional abandonment and physical pain—had been braided together for Tommy throughout the rest of his life.

When he was six years old, his mother and father went away to a convention and left him with an aunt and uncle who were very strict and rigid. He was miserable the first day and ended up "accidentally" running his bike into a tree. His parents had to come home early to take him to a specialist. When he was eight, he was taking a rock-climbing course. A bully in the group started picking on him. In an attempt to get away from his antagonist, Tommy slipped and fell ten feet, sustaining a head injury. Later, he sprained his ankle at camp after his first real girlfriend rejected him. His broken wrist happened when he went skiing right after breaking up with another girlfriend. At eighteen, he thought he had found the girl he wanted to marry, only to discover that she was cheating on him. He got on his motorcycle and rode as fast as he could and ended up having the most serious accident of his life!

In college, he fell in love again. This time when a breakup occurred, he didn't have an accident. Instead, he ate! While that might seem at first to be a departure from his pattern of accidents, it was simply a transfer of that same destructive energy to another habit—overeating. Even though gaining twenty pounds was not an accident, it was still an unconscious act, and a self-destructive one at that.

For the first time in his life, Tommy realized how his hidden feelings were actually controlling his life. He admitted to being a little spooked by the whole discovery, but he knew in the long run that this new-found knowledge would help him make better decisions. He had always thought his accidents were just that—accidents—and not anything that he had any hand in creating. He'd been curious about why he'd been overeating so much in the last few years, but he told Linda that he would have never connected that to his relationship problems, let alone his tricycle accident when he was four years old!

The next time Tommy and his then current girlfriend experienced some difficulties in their relationship, Tommy watched his own behavior more closely than he had in the past. He was able to recognize his exaggerated fear of abandonment and how he used food to hide that fear. Instead of falling back into his old habit of overeating during times of emotional stress, he booked a session with Linda where he allowed himself to experience and express the vulnerability he felt at the possibility of another failed relationship. As he let himself feel what was really going on instead of distracting himself with activity (initially as the baby-sitter encouraged and later as he did by skiing and riding his motorcycle and overeating), he was gradually able to circumvent his unconscious and automatic tendency to overeat.

Linda says that when she last saw Tommy, he had been enjoying a successful relationship with another young woman for eighteen months and was preparing to propose to her. He had maintained his weight and suffered no physical injuries during that time. He had learned how to recognize and assess his feelings and express them appropriately, instead of letting them sabotage his positive self-image.

As you complete your graph and add your emotional information, your pattern may not be as evident as Tommy's. If you look more closely, however, and allow your memory and information from your relatives to fill in any blank spots in your history, you may find as Tommy did that unresolved feelings are the culprit with which you need to deal.

Understanding why you do something and then not doing it again are two distinctly different things. Also, the job of maintaining your new self-image may be a bigger issue than the initial change itself. If you find yourself getting stuck in those old habits once again, remember Charlie, Sarah, and Tommy. They found their answers beneath the surface of their behavior. When those deeper issues were resolved, food and eating relaxed into a more gentle focus in their lives. We are confident that can happen for you as well.

21

When Food No Longer Controls Your Life

If food has been a controlling factor throughout your life, you probably can't imagine living without it. In fact, it may well be the central focus of your existence. If that's the case, it may be hard for you to believe that millions of people live every day without giving food much thought at all. They enjoy eating, of course, but it's just one of their many pleasures, instead of the only one!

We've shared with you case histories of people who have discovered how to enjoy food without allowing it to run their lives. For every one of them, it took moving out of the dark realm of denial into the light-filled world of awareness. It took patience, time, and energy, and it took giving up the myths of quick and easy solutions. They all had to come down from their own moon palaces. They all agree, however, that their lives feel and work better now than ever before. They say the trials and tribulations were worth the outcome.

Ricardo

"I never realized I was basing so much of my life on food and my next meal. I'm an artist and even though I have always been able to lose myself in my craft, my most satisfying moments were when I was eating the most delicious meals I could find. Many times as I painted by myself, I would visualize the food I would be sharing with friends later that evening. That meal would be the highlight of my day. I spent an inordinate amount of time finding just the right place to eat, getting reservations, and making sure my friends could join me there. I also spent a lot of money. I hate to admit it, but I was a food snob. My friends gave me a hard time about that, but I claimed I just liked to eat exquisite food. That was true. But in all honesty, finding the 'right meal' had become a daily obsession.

"My wake-up call came from Yvette, a young woman I'd started dating. Yvette had once been anorexic and was therefore intimately familiar with food obsessions. Looking back, I can see now that she chose her words carefully when she began to confront me on my eating habits.

"In those days, the only meal I ate was dinner, and then I really gorged myself. Most of the time, Yvette and I didn't start eating until seven or eight in the evening, and the meal—complete with the perfect wine and dessert—often didn't end until ten or eleven o'clock. I was never hungry in the morning, and so I would drink coffee all day while I painted and, of course, planned my next fabulous meal.

"I was so attracted to Yvette that when she seduced me one afternoon, I actually forgot my ritual of planning my evening meal. We were at her house and she brought out some fruit and cheese for a dinner snack and then we made love all through the night.

"The next morning, we were starving (a sensation I'd not felt for years at that hour of the day). We went out and had breakfast and while we were eating, Yvette began telling me about her experiences of getting back on track after having spent so many years anorexic. She talked about learning the importance of eating small amounts of food throughout the day and avoiding large heavy meals. She educated me about what was happening inside my body when I would eat so much and then go home to bed. We talked about the habit I had gotten into of isolating myself all day and then socializing every evening at dinner. I began to understand what it was that I wanted, what the obsession was all about. It was being with my friends to share my intense pleasure of eating. Most of the time, I ended up paying for the entire meal. 'When you are treating them all the time, how do you know they are really your friends?' Yvette asked. She made a good point!

"She also talked about something she had learned in her recovery—that what you focus on expands. *What you focus on expands.* That simple phrase became a turning point in my life. I had been focusing on food and unconsciously 'buying' the attention of my friends because I didn't want to eat by myself and I didn't think they would join me if I didn't foot the bill. What would happen if I ate three times a day and had something else to do besides traipse all over New York City looking for my next food fix? I was intrigued with that possibility.

"I have to admit that at first I substituted Yvette for my friends. Because of her history, she had an interest in helping me, so I accepted her direction. She and I lived together off and on for six months. During that time, I learned how to eat three meals a day. We went out for lunch, so I still got my 'fix' of fine meals (for a lot less money, I might add), and she taught me how to cook simple, delicious dinners in my apartment. We started eating at six o'clock, skipped the dessert, and didn't eat again until breakfast the next day.

"The true friends I had (that is, those who weren't simply leeching off me for meals) still came around. One time, Yvette suggested I ask them to bring something to share for an evening meal instead of going out with them. What a change in lifestyle!

"There were other unexpected benefits to this new way of being. Among them was the fact that my creative work was much better. That was because I no longer had a dual focus of painting and eating. Now, all my energy could go into my art without visions of food floating before my eyes! Even when Yvette wasn't around, I began going out to lunch by myself. I felt less isolated in my work when I took a break for lunch and rejoined the human race. Food began to take a normal place in my life. I got a new agent and my work really took off.

"After several months of a great relationship, Yvette joined a traveling dance troupe and we eventually lost contact. When I look back at that time, I still think of her as an angel. That was two years ago and since that time, my food obsession has vanished and my next meal no longer controls my life. I still enjoy good food, but it is just one of the many experiences in life that I enjoy. I don't think a day goes by that I don't remember that *what you focus on expands*. Thank you, Yvette, wherever you are!"

Ricardo had a little help from a friend. Remember, the first step out of denial into awareness often comes from observing someone else. But it can also come from just honoring your own needs and wants.

Andy

Andy had been a very happy and popular cheerleader in high school. She had a host of friends and dates and was looking forward to graduation. Just for fun, she wanted to take a year off between high school and college and be a ski instructor. It was a dream not shared by her parents, however. They insisted she start college immediately after high school.

Andy obliged, but once she was in college, she was no longer the happy-go-lucky girl she was in high school. She found herself the proverbial little fish in a big pond, and she was hopelessly homesick. When she begged her parents to come get her and take her home, their response was, "No way! You just got there. Focus on your studies. You'll be fine." She felt abandoned, out of touch, and totally out of control of her life. There was one thing she could control, however, and that was what she ate. She chose to barely eat at all. She began measuring out every small morsel of food she allowed herself. She felt proud of her ability to manipulate her appetite and was quite proud of the skinny body she was creating.

When Andy went home for the holidays, her sister was shocked at how emaciated she looked. Still, no one really interceded other than to encourage her to eat, which of course, she didn't. Her first year in college was absolutely miserable and her anorexia grew worse with every passing day. Just before the end of that first school year, her roommate and friends confronted her and "escorted" her to the school counselor. That was when Andy began learning about her own needs and wants.

Andy told the counselor about her dream of being a ski instructor, about her loneliness, and how she felt so small and insignificant in such a big school. The counselor focused on her strengths, which were many, and the strong support of her friends. She gradually guided Andy out of denial and into the awareness of how dangerous her eating disorder had become. Even though Andy was irritated that her friends had revealed her eating habits to the counselor, she was also relieved. Somebody cared after all!

With the unwavering support of both the counselor and her friends, Andy began the process of eating small bites every few hours. Over a period of a few months, she gently increased her food intake and she eventually gained the weight she had lost in that first year of college.

Even though Andy continued to eat a healthy diet and remained in school, she was never completely happy with her college experience. She did what it took, however, to get through it and with good grades. On the day of graduation, she packed her car and drove straight to Colorado and got a job as a ski instructor! Her parents were unhappy with that decision, but she was on her own now and so they no longer had any financial hold on her. Andy says that the three years she worked in Colorado were some of the happiest times of her life. She was doing what she absolutely wanted to do, when she wanted to do it, and with whom she wanted to do it!

Although she'd already learn to eat well before graduating from college, she says she knows that those few years in Colorado were the turning point in her life. It was then, when she was beyond the confines of college and no longer dependent on her parents, that she was finally able to take complete control of her life and when that happened, her natural appetite and regular eating habits fell into place.

Linda has known Andy for seven years and has watched her go through good times and bad. Not once has she seen Andy return to her old habit of withholding food from herself as a means of controlling her life. By receiving support and focusing on her dream, she was able to free herself from a deadly pattern. She was lucky. Most people who suffer from anorexia have a much more difficult time breaking the hold of this destructive disease.

Josie

"I don't have any friends and I'm bored!" Josie told Linda in their first therapy session. "All I do is work and watch television. I hate this town—everyone is so unfriendly. My only form of pleasure is overeating and even though I hate the way my body looks, I don't want to give up eating the way I want to. It's the only thing I have to look forward to." Josie was trapped. As is the case with so many people, food was her only companion. It was the only thing that she felt gave her pleasure.

As part of Josie's therapy, Linda gave her an assignment. She was to come back to her next session with a list of ten things she liked to do for fun, besides watching television and movies. Although she only came up with five, that was a start. Her next assignment was to actually do one of those five things on her list. She chose to take dance lessons at a nearby studio. Even though she'd never had dance lessons, Josie proved to be very light on her feet. She also enjoyed herself and while there met another young woman who was also lonely. Josie and her new friend ventured out into the city and went to museums, free concerts, and lots of happy hours at bars where they could practice dancing. Without realizing it, Josie had greatly increased her level of physical activity (she'd been almost completely sedentary before), and started losing weight. She was so busy playing that she barely noticed!

She went from dance lessons to joining a singles club to taking ice skating lessons to roller-blading. In the beginning, she tended to do too much because she'd felt so deprived of fun and companionship for nearly all her life. Eventually, she discovered what she liked to do the best and balanced her socializing, other activities, and work. Josie, the woman who had at first described herself as bored, was now happily occupied with all the fun events that had always been there but she'd never noticed.

Boredom can blind you, blocking you from seeing your options. Once you see all the different things life has to offer, it is almost impossible to be bored again. Josie now knew another way of being, and in choosing balanced activity instead of allowing herself to be smothered in boredom, she was able to let food relax into its proper place in the background of her life. Through the years, Josie still occasionally fell back into her old negative beliefs of boredom, but only for a day or two at a time. She knows from her new experiences that boredom is just a state of mind. Now she knows exactly who controls her mind. She does!

What would your life look like if you weren't thinking about food and eating so much (or so little)? What is it that you want more than anything? To be more athletic? More attractive or creative? To get a better job or perhaps to change occupations altogether? Do you desire a romantic relationship? Freeing yourself of being controlled by food doesn't guarantee any of your desires will come true, but it will free up your energy and make it possible for you to work on the real issues that have been blocking you from realizing your dreams. Whether you are eating at home, with relatives who substitute food for love, or in a restaurant, there is a life beyond being controlled by your desire or fear of food and it's time to begin living it!

22

Help! I'm Eating Out! What Do I Do?

You've made a commitment to honor your body and you're already seeing some progress. So how do you maintain that commitment in the midst of everyday interruptions and challenges? We will help you discover how to do that. You will learn how empowering it is to be in control of the circumstances of your life.

The times during which we deviate from our normal routines present us with opportunities for growth and for stretching ourselves by discarding all our old excuses. At times such as these, we should not feel embarrassed about ourselves, but rather we should use them to make different choices and to learn new behaviors and thoughts that build us up rather than tear us down. When you backslide (or otherwise deviate from your plan) you must learn to recognize it as a gift of learning. If you'll only take the time to look, you'll discover pearls of wisdom about yourself that you've probably kept buried inside. It's important for you to know that the unconscious negative thoughts that will undoubtedly arise when you backslide have been there all along. Backsliding is your opportunity to see them, learn about them, change them, and then heal.

Social outings, dining out, traveling, busy schedules—these are all things that can trigger backsliding and negative thoughts about ourselves. These events are usually loaded with emotions that are neither necessarily good nor bad, but are simply signals from our inner wisdom telling us that something is different and that we need to pay attention.

In her practice, Kathleen teaches people how to stay conscious and prepare for these events. When you're getting ready to go out on a dinner date or to the theatre, for example, you take great care in choosing what clothes and jewelry you will wear, how your hair is done and your nails are manicured, etc. Then why not take the same care in preparing your thoughts for the same event? Kathleen says the best way she's found to stay conscious about an event and what her behavior will be in regard to any food that's served there is to ask herself some simple questions beforehand. She suggests taking the time to write your answers down in your journal and to then devise a plan. Being armed with a plan and a more conscious view of the event, she says, will reap a multitude of benefits.

Here are some questions you might want to ask yourself about an upcoming trip or wedding, office party, or whatever social event finds you having to eat away from home:

- **Why are you going?** Is it an obligation? Is it for fun? Is it to reconnect with friends or family you haven't seen for a while?

- **What does this bring up for you?** When you are clear about why you are going, many times different emotions arise. Seeing these before you go helps you to deal with them and not to use food to cover them over.

- **What kind of food will be served there?** If possible, decide before getting there what your choices will be. Then you can go more focused on the event than on the food.

- **How will you support your body during the event?** Will you have had nutrient-dense food before going to the event? Are you going with an empty and growling stomach? An empty stomach is usually another setup for overeating. It is not only good to look at food choices, but also the energy that will be required of you during the event. Do you need extra sleep beforehand or afterwards? If so, do you need to clear your calendar to make sure this happens? Often dragging oneself around for days after an event is a setup for overeating the wrong types of food. When we're worn out, we'll grab anything just to bring our energy level back up.

- **How will you relate to alcohol?** If alcohol presents a problem for you, thinking of how you will relate ahead of time will help you to stay focused. If drinking alcohol is not a problem and you enjoy a glass of wine once in a while, then how much will you have? Will you drink on an empty stomach?

Peter

Peter came to see Kathleen prior to going to an event at a local restaurant. His answers to these questions may help you see the benefit in such an exercise as the one described above. He was willing to learn how to ask himself these questions because he wanted help, for he admitted that restaurants were the basis of his entire social life and that he often ate and drank too much. Here are his answers:

- **Why are you going?** "I am going because I love being with these people and it's fun. Secondly, I love the food at this restaurant."

- **What does this bring up for you?** "The laughter, fun, good company, and great food are just pure pleasure."

- **What kind of food will be served there?** "Usually, we start with cocktails and appetizers and move on to gourmet entrees with wine and then coffee and dessert and maybe after-dinner drinks. It keeps the evening going in a slow, leisurely pace."

- **How will you support your body during this event?** "I'm still unclear as to how I will support my body. But I will not have had 'nutrient-dense food' beforehand because I want to leave room for the rich meal and dessert and all the rest."

- **How will you relate to alcohol?** "This is a hard one because I do not want to be perceived as different. I don't want to call attention to myself. I want to enjoy the food and drink I love and not feel deprived. But I also don't want to feel bad the next day after eating and drinking like I usually do. Then I feel tired and irritable and disappointed with myself that I could not stick to my commitment and plan. But I do not want a good time to turn into a struggle."

When Peter reviewed his answers, he saw how he was setting himself up to repeat the same old behaviors once again. The new insight he gained was that he didn't like what he'd been doing, but neither did he want to draw attention to himself by being different nor did he want to feel deprived.

Some Suggestions If You Find Yourself in a Similar Situation

Get a good night's sleep the night before the event. Your body can handle the fun and food better when it is rested. Drink plenty of water and eat lightly during the day of the event. Eat fruits and vegetables and simple proteins (such as eggs or tofu) at the last meal prior to the event. Before going to the restaurant, assess your hunger. If you are starving, have a couple of almonds, an apple, a piece of turkey, or some carrots before you go.

When you get to the restaurant, the first thing they do is take your order for drinks and then they usually place a basket of bread on the table. Instead of eating the bread and drinking a cocktail, order a small appetizer of some nutritious food (nothing fried). Wait until you've eaten your appetizer before you start to drink any alcohol. And instead of ordering a second cocktail, ask for some sparkling water with a lemon or lime wedge, and then continue drinking the water with your meal. If you'd prefer, have them serve the water in a wine glass.

Order your entrée and instead of a side order of potato, pasta, or rice, ask for extra steamed vegetables. This way, you are cutting down on the foods that make you feel heavy and bloated. After dinner, skip the coffee and drink some hot tea which, as pointed out in Chapter Eight, contains about half the caffeine that coffee does. If you want dessert, see if someone is willing to split it with you. If not, ask for another plate and cut your dessert in half and ask the waiter to remove the other half from the table. Now enjoy every bite of your dessert! Before you decide to have that after-dinner drink, assess how full you are. If you decide to have a drink, which one will be the least filling? Will it make you feel groggy the next day? Ask yourself if you wouldn't be happier in the long run if you simply had some more sparkling water.

If you take the time to think and plan ahead for the event, you will quickly begin making better choices for yourself. Remember, no one is saying no to you. We often get in a rebellious frame of mind and become bound and determined to do whatever we darned well please, especially if we think someone is saying we can't or shouldn't have something. That worked well as a child when we were trying to gain our independence. But as adults, we sometimes still act as though to eat properly is like our parents shaking their finger at us and saying no to the things we want.

Do we really want food that is depleting us day in and day out? You are the adult making choices that honor and support your body. You are saying no to tiredness, stiff joints, headaches, irritability, low self-esteem, and the many other aches and pains and diseases that can arise from making poor food choices. If you stop and ask yourself the questions before an event as Peter did, you will be surprised how many times that little kid comes up to you and says, "You can't tell me what I can and cannot have!" Health and vitality depends upon your ability to recognize that inner voice and then reassuring your little kid inside that you are making choices to feel good and it will not be deprived.

Going to a Friend's or Relative's House for Dinner

These situations can be tricky. For one thing, you don't have the same control of the menu as you do at a restaurant. Here is an example from Leah's situation. It is her grandmother's birthday. Leah loves seeing her grandma. Grandma always insists on cooking even on her special day, so the whole family is heading over there for dinner. Two days earlier, Leah had gotten into an argument with her father over an investment she'd made and he'd told her that she'd made a stupid mistake. She'd not spoken to him since. She knows, of course, that he will be at her grandma's birthday party.

- **Why are you going?** "I am going because I love Grandma and I want to help her celebrate her birthday. She's getting up there in years, but she's healthy. I'm glad I still have the opportunity to do this."

- **What does this bring up for you?** "Joy in celebrating with Grandma, but anger at seeing my dad. He is controlling and demeaning whenever I don't see things his way. He makes me feel inadequate and small."

- **What kind of food will be served there?** "Well, Grandma is a meat, potato, and gravy lover. We might have some canned peas, but probably no other vegetables. She always serves the same sweet white wine and we use it to toast with and drink with our meal. For dessert, there is always chocolate cake with fudge icing. It's my favorite and Grandma has always made it for me. It brings back memories of good times with lots of love and acceptance." (Note: Thinking about this makes Leah realize that she does not feel accepted by her father and the cake could trigger overeating to cover over these feelings.)

- **How will you support your body during this event?** "I am going to eat lightly throughout the day, since the meal is going to be heavy. I plan on having fruit and two scrambled eggs for breakfast and for lunch, a large vegetable salad and some vegetable soup. I also plan to drink even more water than I normally do so that my body will be well hydrated in order to help digest and flush the fat-laden meal I know Grandma will be serving." (Note: Leah also ate a small handful of almonds before going so she wouldn't be hungry when she got there. She reported that this way, she was able to think through her portions more consciously. She decided she would eat the chocolate cake and really enjoy it, but she would limit herself to one piece and would savor every bite and eat it slowly. She was going to eat it feeling the love from her grandmother. Although she wouldn't cover up the feelings with her father, she didn't feel as though this was the appropriate time and place to work out a lifetime of issues with him.)

- **How will you relate to the alcohol being served?** "I'll admit to liking sweet wine with my meals. However, by looking over what I've written in my journal, I realized that the wine makes it difficult for me to have a good night's sleep and it usually gives me a headache the next day. I've decided to have one glass and toast Grandma during dinner. Other than that, I plan to drink water with my dinner.

Let's take another example. You are going to be with friends to watch the Super Bowl and you know the menu is going to consist of chips, beer, and pizza. Start asking yourself the questions we suggested until you have a plan for yourself and are clear about why it is that you're going. You are not going just to eat. You are going to be with friends and enjoy the game. Be focused and conscious of what you are doing. Your plan might be to eat a salad and a chicken breast before going. When you get there, your plan might be to have two beers, a couple of handfuls of chips, and two pieces of pizza. You will have decided ahead of time to eat slowly and make your food stretch throughout the game. You will drink water in between eating.

You are in charge, so get creative with your plan. The more you think through what you are going to do and eat, the more powerful you will feel and the easier the issue of food will become. Remember that your main intention is to have health, clarity of thought, and vitality. Always be grateful to your body for how well it responds to your new and responsible approach to eating. In the end, your feelings of renewed good health will be a continual motivating factor.

Travel

This is the ultimate challenge for most of our clients, especially those who have to travel extensively. Again, if you take the time to ask yourself the questions above, they will help you focus on the travel time and to make choices regarding how you will relate to it. Here are some suggestions:

- On the day you travel, bring with you a small, insulated lunch bag packed with nutritious food. This way, you will not be caught hungry with only fast food or airline fare as a choice.

- Drink more water than you normally do—at least an additional two glasses a day. Traveling (especially air travel) is dehydrating to the body.

- Eat smaller meals than you usually do at home. Your body is under a stressful situation because there is change. Do not make it work harder to digest large portions of food.

- Eat simple foods in their natural state. For instance, eat more green salads and fruit throughout the day. Eat easy-to-digest proteins such as fish, eggs, chicken, turkey, or tofu. Stay away from fried, greasy foods and foods with cream sauces.

- Bless all food before eating. This is helpful before any meal, but especially when you're traveling. Think of all the people and animals and the earth that are responsible for providing this food. Be grateful for their contributions. Earlier, we talked about the energy and vibration of food. A blessing always helps raise the vibration of the food, which in turn brings better health to you. Consider a blessing in which you ask that the vibration of your food be raised to serve your highest good and then give thanks for all who have been involved in bringing it to you.

Busy Schedules

Crammed agendas have become routine for a lot of us. Our hurried lifestyles make it easy to offer excuses as we push through the day putting into our mouth whatever is close at hand and convenient. These times not only make digestion more difficult, but they also challenge our adrenal glands and immune systems—harried times cause our bodies to become depleted more easily.

Now more than ever, our bodies need nutrition without having to digest large quantities of food. Eating is best kept to such simple foods as fruits and vegetables and simple proteins and complex carbohydrates (as discussed in Part II). Before you start your week, ask yourself these questions and record your answers in your journal:

- **Is this project that has me so busy worth my health and peace of mind?**

- **How do I want to relate to food this week?** Do I shop ahead of time and have foods prepared and ready for the week? Are there healthy restaurant choices close by in case I need a quick bite? When the office is sending out for lunch, what choices will I make?

- **Do I have a system set up for myself to make sure I'm drinking enough water?** One possible solution is to have a 24-ounce glass of water on your desk and drink two to three of these during the workday.

- **Am I getting adequate sleep?** If you're dragging, it's hard to stay focused on the task at hand, let alone a food plan.

- **Am I moving my body?** Note: Just simple motion every hour is helpful. Take the stairs instead of the elevator, stretch, do jumping jacks, go for a walk during your lunch hour. Give your body the movement it needs to function properly. Be creative and come up with fun ways to move.

If we're not taking care of ourselves, it's obvious that we will not have a lot to offer to our jobs, to our fellow workers, to our families and friends, or most of all to ourselves. Despite the fact that these are challenging times, every positive thought and action will produce more clarity, feelings of self worth, creativity, energy, and personal power. When you're in this flow, you are a joy to yourself and everyone around you!

All of the events we discussed in this chapter are opportunities for growth and change, even if you don't follow our suggestions to the letter. What we do ask is that you take note of what happened and to be conscious of your feelings and behavior. Most importantly, take responsibility for your actions. Life is all about choices, and choosing to make excuses only keeps you stuck. Use these events to move your life forward. Don't squander precious life energy beating yourself up. Life is a journey that you should allow to propel you forward. Staying in the past to punish yourself is a waste of energy. Learn, be thankful for the experience, and move forward. You will be wise and more powerful. If ever you stray from your plan, stop to laugh at yourself. And then simply return to your intent to be healthy, vibrant with clarity of mind, and go on. You are getting better everyday!

23

Can I Ever Eat the Foods I Love?

This chapter will be short. Why? Because there are no forbidden foods! We can have whatever we want. It is the consciousness of what we are thinking and feeling about the food that is important. It is staying open to our inner wisdom inside and not the scolding parent.

The child in us wants that donut and defies anyone to tell us that it's not good for us. When you find yourself in this place of rebellion, it is usually the child within that is responding to the scolding parent. When you see the donut and consciously decide you're going to eat it and enjoy every bite, it removes the rebellion from clouding the issue of the donut. After you've eaten the donut, you can decide to listen to your body and see how it reacted to the donut. Did you feel really satisfied? Did you feel guilty? Did you feel bloated and stuffed? Did you feel tired shortly after eating it? Did this food bring you joy and vitality, or did it leave you feeling depleted? Listen and let your body guide you.

It is the contrast of different foods and how our body reacts to them that provides us with growth opportunities. Many times, we eat quickly what we deem "forbidden foods" so that we don't even know that we've eaten them. Have you ever had a package of M&M's disappear and you don't even remember eating them? Kathleen admits to this.

"When I started to eat more consciously, I didn't stop eating M&M's. Instead, I would just eat three at a time and thoroughly enjoy them. After about fifteen to twenty, I would stop and put the bag away. I felt great and did not get the usual groggy feeling I would have when I used to eat the whole bag. The bonus? I had more M&M's left for the next day!" As time went on, however, she started to wonder why she felt she needed to treat herself every day. She followed her own advice and began keeping notes in her journal.

"What I discovered with time was that I felt as though I gave a lot to others during the day and didn't know how to receive what it was that I needed. I began to realize that people did try to do things for me, but that I never trusted them or their motives. Therefore, I never felt loved by their behavior. I didn't believe I was lovable or that I deserved pleasure and happiness. All of this insight from just writing about some M&M's!

"Seeing this started me on a journey of learning to love myself and trusting that I am loved just because I am. Every time I felt like I needed a treat, I would ask myself what it was that I wasn't letting in. What gift was waiting for me? What love and joy were there for me and were the M&M's going to cover it? I slowly gained the insight that these treats were my way of shutting out others and thus the possibility of a fuller and more meaningful life. Once I began to open up and be more receptive to the love of others, I found I could easily decide if I wanted the treat or not. It is never an issue of whether or not I can or should have it. Learning to trust was a lesson that took me several years to learn. Throughout it all, food was always a helpful indicator where I was in the process."

Being in balance and in tune with herself paid an unexpected dividend when her very fit and healthy husband woke up one day and could hardly walk. "His legs were swollen, very hard, and cold. He was taken straight to the emergency room where it was determined that a large blood clot extended from his chest all the way down past both of his knees. He was given blood thinners for two weeks, but his condition worsened and emergency surgery was ordered. The surgeon told Kathleen that his first job was to try to save her husband's life, and only then to attempt to save his legs and kidneys. They wheeled him away and Kathleen was left by herself.

"Usually, I would have been in a panic. In the past, I only felt secure if I had all my options worked out beforehand. Now everything important in my life was out of my control. What happened that day was very different. I automatically realized my husband and I were both loved. This was true, even if he died. Whatever happened was the best for both of us. I became so peaceful and started to be grateful for all we'd had together and what a gift our relationship was.

"In the middle of the operation, the surgeon came out to report to me that everything was going as well as could be expected, but there were no certainties. He seemed concerned that I was so calm. I looked him in the eye and told him I understood what was going on, but that I was choosing to trust. As it turned out, my husband not only lived, but three surgeries and many close calls later, he is now running and hiking and doing all the things he used to do. The doctors are baffled.

"My husband gained his own insights from all of this; but for me, I realized that by being conscious and in touch with my inner wisdom, I was in a good and whole place in my life. I was worthy and I was loved".

Kathleen came to realize that by taking responsibility for her life in that small area that controlled how she ate M&M's, she'd opened an area that had been blocked for many years. "Staying conscious to my life led me to a place of peace and happiness nothing can take from me, not even the threat of death."

That is real power. It is available to us all.

Tips for Staying on the Path

You do have the power. By reading this book, you've exercised some of the power needed to make the changes you desire in your body and in your life. Our guess is that you've already experienced the joy of some successes—and also that you've endured the disappointment of a few failures—along the way. Occasional failures are part of the process. It's important for you to know that and to know that you can forgive yourself and keep moving forward.

We've compiled some suggestions that will help you continue on the path of making peace with your body, connecting with your spirit and your feelings, and of having a *Full Heart/Satisfied Belly*! Return to these whenever you feel as though you may have temporarily lost direction.

- Learn which activities bring you inner quiet, peace, and wisdom. Repeat these experiences frequently, especially whenever you find yourself being concerned about how you look to others.

- Remind yourself to have patience. Personal growth is a steady and ongoing process, not something you can pop into a microwave. Develop tolerance for yourself and for your wonderful journey of transformation.

- For heaven's sake, stop scaring yourself with negative words and thoughts about how you look and feel!

- Learn to identify the feeling of satisfaction in your body and then set a goal to experience that feeling at least once a day.

- When you find yourself craving something, distract yourself for fifteen minutes and see if you still want it at the end of that time.

- When you catch yourself making "automatic pilot" decisions about what to eat, stop and recommit to making healthy lifestyle and food choices.

- Did you find yourself eating because you were tired? Take some time to rest. Were you eating because you were sad or angry? Learn to express your feelings appropriately.

- What are you really hungry for? Be honest with yourself, for it may not be food that you want.

- Tell someone you trust about what you have been eating.

- Get support when attempting to stop compulsive behavior.

- Feed yourself and your family organic food.

- Keep a food journal for at least thirty days.

- As much as possible, avoid highly processed foods and junk foods.

- Drink a minimum of half your body weight in ounces of water each day.

- For at least twenty minutes every day, walk or do some other form of physical exercise.

- Honor your body's request for rest.

- Dedicate fifteen minutes a day to prayer or meditation.

- Remember to feed your conscious and subconscious mind with positive thoughts.

Most importantly, learn to listen to your body and heed its messages. It wants what's best for you, too!

Suggested Reading

Ballentine, Rudolph, M.D. *Radical Healing, Integrating the World's Great Therapeutic Traditions to Create a New Transformative Medicine,* Three Rivers Press, New York, New York, 1999 http://www.radicalhealing.com/

Ballentine introduces the principles of holistic healing and presents an integrated system combining the awareness, tools, and practices taught by a variety of healing disciplines, including Ayurveda, homeopathy, and herbal medicine. Ballentine explains the principles of "nature's medicinals," based on the herbal traditions of China, India (Ayurvedic), Europe, and Native America. He presents several self-assessment techniques, including body maps and mind/body types. He describes the use of exercise, nutrition and cleansing (detoxification), and holistic techniques for working with energy and consciousness. Extensive resources for integrating holistic healing approaches into your daily life let you continue after the book ends.

Capodilupo, Linda, *Thin Through the Power of Spirit,* DeVorss, Marina del Rey, California, 1999

Capodilupo makes the startling disclosure that excessive overweight is a spiritual problem, the root cause of which lies in the mind. The seriously overweight person is subconsciously unhappy with, and warring against, their own physical incarnation. With this perception that the "soul" or self is caught in the fleshy prison of the body, the compulsion to overeat takes over—a symbolic acting-out of this imprisonment. It shows the readers how to change their world view, psychology, body image, and food choices so that they can move out of the prison of excess weight and into conditions of normal weight and increased freedom.

Critser, Greg, *Fat Land, How Americans Became the Fattest People in the World*, Houghton Mifflin Company, Boston & New York, 2003

Critser details what happened as a river of corn syrup (and cheap, lardlike palm oil) met with a fast-food marketing strategy that prized sales-via super-sized "value" meals-over quality or conscience. The surgeon general has declared obesity an epidemic. About 61% of Americans are now overweight 20% of us are obese. Type 2 (i.e., fat-related) diabetes is exploding, even among children. Critser's book vividly describes the physical suffering that comes from being fat. The author shows how the poor become the fattest victimized above all by the lack of awareness. In vivid prose conveying the urgency of the situation, with just the right amount of detail for general readers,

Gerber, Richard, M.D., *Vibrational Medicine, New Choices for Healing Ourselves*, Bear & Company, Santa Fe, New Mexico 1988

Vibrational remedies don't contain a substance that promotes healing—they contain the "signature" or vibration of a particular substance. That vibration resonates with the vibration of human cells to stimulate healing. Many people have tried vibrational remedies and know they work. Gerber's provides the scientific data needed to validate that knowledge. It is a treasure trove of information; and those who have experienced it first hand will appreciate the thoroughness of his research and documentation..

Hirschmann, Jane R. and Munter, Carol H., *When Women Stop Hating Their Bodies*, Ballantine Books, New York, New York 1995 http://www.overcomingovereating.com/
Munter and Hirschmann call this syndrome "Bad Body Fever" and demonstrate how "bad body thoughts" are clues to our emotional lives. They explore the difficulties women encounter replacing dieting with demand feeding. And finally, they teach us how to think about our problems rather than eat about them—so that food can resume its proper place in our lives.

Roth, Geneen, *Why Weight? A Guide To Ending Compulsive Eating*, Penguin Books, New York, New York 1989

After Feeding the Hungry Heart and Breaking Free from Compulsive Eating, Roth offers a workbook that will enable readers to explore for themselves the issues that lead to compulsive eating

Migliore, Marilyn, *The Hunger Within*, Doubleday, New York, New York 1998 http://www.weightfocus.com/focus_faculty.asp?f=weight_gain&b=weightfocus&d=migliore_marilyn

This concrete, lucid, step-by-step guide explores the core reasons that lead to overeating, identifies the triggers that precipitate bingeing, and breaks the vicious cycle of yo-yo dieting.

Virtue, Doreen Ph.D., *Constant Craving*, Hay House, Carlsbad, California 1995

Why do we crave chocolate? Potato chips? Cheeseburgers? Ice cream? According to author Doreen Virtue, "we intuitively crave foods that perfectly match our emotional needs, and that there are many psychoactive (mood-altering) properties in the food we eat." This fun book provides information that everyone who enjoys eating will find interesting.

Wilde, Stuart, *Weight Loss for the Mind,* Hay House, Carlsbad, CA 1994

Wilde teaches readers how to deal with opinions, feelings, contradiction, expectancy, and finally how to elevate your spirits to feel freer and lighter.

www.weightwatchers.com

www.overeatersanonymous.com

References

Chapter Six

Hartmann, Thom, *The Last Hours of Ancient Sunlight*, Mythical Books, Northfield, Vermont 1998

Hawken, Paul, *The Ecology of Commerce*, Harper Business, New York, NY, 1993

Robbins, John, *Diet For A New America*, H J Kramer, Tiburon, CA 1987

Teitel, Martin, Ph.D. and Wilson, Kimberly, *Genetically Engineered Food: Changing the Nature of Nature*, Park Street Press, Rochester, Vermont, 1999

Winter, Ruth, M.S., *Poisons In Your Food*, Crown Publishers, Inc., New York, NY 1991

Chapter Eight

Blaylock, Russell L., M.D., *Excitotoxins, The Taste That Kills*, Health Press, Sante Fe, New Mexico, 1997

DesMaisons, Kathleen, Ph.D., *Potatoes not Prozac*, Simon & Schuster, New York, NY, 1998

Santillo, Humbart, N.D., *Intuitive Eating*, Hohm Press, Prescott, AZ, 1993

Schlosser, Eric, *Fast Food Nation*, Houghton Mifflin Company, Boston, 2001

Tips, Jack, ND, Ph.D., CCN, *The Weight Is Over*, Apple-A-Day Enterprises, Inc., 1999

Chapter Nine

Duncan, Lindsey, C.N., *Healthy And Natural Journal, Internal Detoxification.*

Jensen, Bernard, Ph.D., *The Chemistry of Man*, Bernard Jensen International, Escondido, CA 1983

Weil Andrew, M.D., *Spontaneous Healing*, Borzoi Books, 1995

Work, Rich, *Proclamations of the Soul*, Asini Publishing, 1999

About the Authors

Kathleen S. Hosner, Ph.D., PA, CT, has practiced in the health care industry for thirty years. She holds a B.S. as a Physician Assistant, an M.S. in Health Services Administration, a Ph.D. in Nutrition, and is a certified colon hydrotherapist. Overcoming her own health challenges led Kathleen to a life of well-being and spiritual purpose. She is passionately committed to teaching her clients and workshop audiences how they, too, can achieve optimal health through becoming aware of their inner wisdom, understanding how the body works, listening to what the body needs, and feeling the connectedness of all life. You can contact Kathleen at <u>khosner@fullbelly.org</u>

Linda Frazee is the founder and president of Positive Imagery, a personal and professional development company based in Scottsdale, Arizona. For the past twenty years, she has assisted individuals, government agencies, nonprofit organizations, small companies, and Fortune 500 firms in redirecting conflicted emotional energy into positive, creative solutions. Linda's organizational consulting takes her throughout the United States. As a national workshop leader and professional speaker, Linda presents personal growth topics to thousands of people each year. She has appeared on television, in commercials, and on national radio to speak on the connection between food and emotions. You can contact Linda at <u>lfrazee@fullbelly.org</u>

**For more information about Full Heart/Satisfied Belly
please visit our website:
www.fullbellyonline.com**

Dr. Hosner and Ms. Frazee offer seminars and workshops that support vibrant health with a wide range of topics:

Corporate Programs: Custom programs available to meet your organizational goals and needs while staying healthy in a stress filled environment.

1. Discover how your body works

2. Learn the link between the food you eat and the mind, body, spirit connection

3. Find freedom from old patterns that keep you locked in destructive behaviors.

4. Learn how to "Make Peace with You Body."

5. Create a simple plan of action to feel better now.

6. Get in touch with your inner guidance

7. Learn to deal effectively with the real issues in your life instead of mediating them with food.

Public Programs: Releasing food obsessions.

1. Discover what you are really craving

2. Learn how to stop compulsive thoughts and behaviors

3. Release old patterns that hold you hostage.

4. End the confusion about "how to eat" and learn the basic truths about the chemistry that governs your body.

5. Create a simple plan of action to support your natural body rhythm and maintain it for life

0-595-31757-X